THE DALAI LAMA AT MIT

THE DALAI LAMA AT MIT

Harvard University Press

Cambridge, Massachusetts / London, England   2006

Edited by Anne Harrington and Arthur Zajonc

Library of Congress Cataloging-in-Publication Data

The Dalai Lama at MIT / edited by Anne Harrington, Arthur
Zajonc.
    p.   cm.
   Records of conference "Investigating the mind," at MIT,
September 2003. Cf. Introduction.
   Includes index.
   ISBN-13: 978-0-674-02319-2 (alk. paper)
   ISBN-10: 0-674-02319-6 (alk. paper)
   1. Psychology and religion—Congresses.   2. Buddhism—
Psychology—Congresses.   I. Bstan-'dzin-rgya-mtsho, Dalai Lama
XIV, 1935–   II. Harrington, Anne, 1960–   III. Zajonc, Arthur.

   BF51.D35 2003
   294.3'3615—dc22   2006041242

To the memory of Francisco Varela

Contents

THE DALAI LAMA AT MIT

I

ORIENTATIONS

Introduction

It was a two-day conference in September 2003, launched under the plain-vanilla title, "Investigating the Mind." The actual opening scene at the meeting, however, was a bit more exotic. Tenzin Gyatso, the fourteenth Dalai Lama of Tibet, sat cross-legged in a comfortable white armchair (shoes set neatly on the floor before him) in the center of a large stage in Kresge Auditorium, on the campus of the Massachusetts Institute of Technology. He had just arrived in Cambridge, Massachusetts, after a flight from Washington, D.C., where he had met with President George W. Bush. However, he said, this meeting at MIT was the most important stop on his three-week North American tour. To the Dalai Lama's left, spread out in a crescent, sat a small group of Buddhist scholars and practitioners, some in standard-issue academic tweeds, some in saffron and orange monastic robes. To his right, in another semicircle, sat a no less carefully selected group of neuroscientists and cognitive scientists. The prominent bouquets of flowers surrounding the Dalai Lama hinted at the high occasion. Otherwise, the arrangements on the stage—the beige carpet, the low-lying tables for laptop computers and bottles of water, the PowerPoint projector—evoked the feel of an academic seminar, or perhaps a scholarly living room chat. If this was the intention, it was a "chat" that was about to take place before a buzzing audience of some 1,200 people: academics, scientists, journalists, Buddhist practitioners, members of the general public, and a smattering of Hollywood celebrities (including the actors Richard Gere and Goldie Hawn). The waiting list of some 1,600 others who had hoped to attend suggested that the organizers could easily have filled a hall the same size again.

What was this meeting all about? What did all who were present— those on stage, the expectant audience, the Dalai Lama himself— imagine they were there to do? When Adam Engle, chairman and cofounder of the Mind and Life Institute, which had organized and largely funded the meeting, stepped up to the podium to welcome the audience, he explained his understanding of the meeting's goals:

Science is the dominant paradigm in modern society for understanding the nature of reality and providing a knowledge base for improving people's lives. Buddhism is a 2,500-year tradition focused on personal liberation, but liberation that is concerned to understand the nature of reality and use that understanding to overcome delusion. So it is the search for a better understanding of the nature of reality that forms the basis for our proposed dialogue between science and Buddhism. Buddhism uses the human mind, refined through meditative practice, as its primary instrument of investigation into the nature of reality. While this method of investigation is based on observation, very rigorous logic, and experimentation, scientists have traditionally viewed it as subjective and at odds with the objectivity of the scientific method.

We believe science is wrong to reject such a mode of investigating the mind, and that there is much potential for fruitful exchange and even active collaborative research between scientists and Buddhists. This meeting has been organized to explore the wisdom and efficacy of this proposal. Our strategy for doing so has been to organize conversations around three topics in psychology that are under active investigation by Western science and to which we believe Buddhism has much to contribute: attention, mental imagery, and emotion.

Later in the meeting, Buddhist scholar Georges Dreyfus would stress that there actually is no such thing as "Buddhism" but only a range of Buddhist perspectives, noting that "Buddhism is a complex and multifaceted tradition that has many mental typologies." Scholars and scientists at this meeting had agreed to focus primarily on perspectives from Tibetan Buddhism, but some future engagement with a larger range of Buddhist perspectives might well be a reasonable desideratum.

Still, even an engagement at this level felt ambitious. And indeed for Engle and the rest of the Mind and Life board, the meeting at MIT was nothing less than a turning point in the history of their organization. The Mind and Life Institute had been founded in the late 1980s as a small, volunteer-run organization dedicated to organizing dialogues between the Dalai Lama and a wide array of scientists. All previous dialogues had taken place in private meetings (with just a handful of invited observers), usually held over the course of five relaxed days at the Dalai Lama's home-in-exile in Dharamsala, India. Though a published volume had resulted from each of the dialogues (see "About the Mind and Life Institute" at the back of this volume), the meetings themselves were not widely publicized and the Mind and Life Institute remained little known. The decision now, in 2003, to "go public" was a gamble. If the meeting failed to impress and engage, Mind and Life's loss of face would be considerable. If it succeeded, the institute would earn the right to call itself a leader in ventures of this sort.

While the Mind and Life Institute may have hoped to position itself as doing something new, the general idea that Buddhism was uniquely well placed to talk constructively with science was more than a century old. Historically, the idea was linked to the rise of a tendency within scientific and scholarly circles to see Christianity as a uniquely *poor* dialogue partner for science. Science could never hope to talk productively with Christianity, it was said, because the two traditions were fundamentally at odds: the one committed to free inquiry and rational explanation, the other to dogmatism and blind faith. The best-known reference point in this hardening position was the impassioned two-volume history written in 1896 by the American educator (and, interestingly, practicing Episcopalian) Andrew Dickson White, *History of the Warfare of Science with Theology in Christendom* (in terms of influence, John Draper's 1874 *Conflict between Science and Religion* ran a close second to White's book).[1]

Against this backdrop, Buddhism—little known to most Western scientists before this time—began to catch at least some people's eye. Though it was a religion, it had no concept of a personal God and no divine Creation story; it seemed broadly compatible with the new Darwinian nontheistic and evolutionary worldview (something that was appreciated by such first-generation Darwinians as Thomas Henry Huxley);[2] it advocated a causal and apparently atomic understanding of all events in the universe (something appreciated by the physicists); and it generally seemed to be remarkably nondogmatic overall. The German-born American philosopher and editor Paul Carus was first exposed to Buddhist thought at the path-breaking 1893 Chicago Parliament of World Religions (which brought together representatives from most world religions for the first time) and never looked back. In an 1896 article entitled "Buddhism and the Religion of Science," he wrote: "Buddha, in so far as we know, is the first positivist, the first humanitarian, the first radical freethinker, the first iconoclast, and the first Prophet of the Religion of Science . . . [He] anticipated even in important details the results of a scientific world-conception."[3]

While most early scientific interest in Buddhism focused on specific areas of apparent compatibility, such as evolutionary theory and atomic theory, the rise of psychology—and, even more, psychotherapy—in the first decades of the twentieth century shifted that focus.

By the mid-twentieth century, it had become increasingly common to see Buddhism as, above all, a theory of mind and human development from which modern Western psychotherapists had much to learn.[4] Various authors argued that Buddhism (and, for some, Eastern mystical traditions in general) offered a way to extend too-narrow Western concepts of selfhood and human development, while promising to reinvigorate the secular work of psychotherapy with new spiritual energy.

Over the years, the Mind and Life Institute had periodically contributed to the therapeutic vision of Buddhism-as-psychology.[5] The vision of dialogue that largely animated the MIT meeting, however, was different. It drew explicitly on the ideas of neuroscientist Francisco Varela and his epistemological and methodological desire to push the "hard science" traditions of cognitive science and neuroscience in new, more radical directions. Well known in neuroscience as the codeveloper, with Humberto Maturana, of the concept of autopoiesis (the idea that living systems are self-organizing entities), Varela founded the Mind and Life Institute with Adam Engle in the late 1980s.[6] Although he died in the spring of 2001 at the age of fifty-four, Varela's intellectual vision of dialogue between cognitive science and Buddhism permeated the MIT meeting. Before his death he penned these words, which are posted on the Mind and Life Web site:

> The natural meeting ground between science and Buddhism is
> . . . at one of the most active research frontiers today. What is involved is learning how to put together the data from the inner examination of human experience with the empirical basis that modern cognitive and affective neuroscience can provide. Such first-person accounts are not a mere "confirmation" of what science can find anyway. [They are] . . . a necessary complement. For instance, unless refined internal descriptions are taken into account in current experiments that use brain imaging to study the neural substrates of emotions or attention, the empirical data cannot be properly interpreted.[7]

Others before Varela had also defended the general proposition that Buddhism offers a way of "inner" knowing that complements or completes the "outer-oriented" approach of Western science. Appealing as such a proposition is, however, some have worried that it encourages a binary style of thinking ("they" are contemplative, "we" are active; "they" are inner-oriented, "we" are externally oriented) that can obscure as much as it illuminates. Tibetologist Donald Lopez has criticized such formulations as symptoms of what he calls "new age orientalism," in which a highly idealized vision of the East (in this case, of Tibetan Buddhism) is held up as a foil to the West, and dialogue or integration between the two traditions is seen as a means of remedying the latter's multiple deficiencies—methodological, ethical, epistemological.[8]

Indeed, during the Mind and Life meeting at MIT some of the scientists on stage would challenge the claim that Western behavioral and brain sciences are all about the "external": these fields, they would note, make regular use of "inner" or "first-person" data, though perhaps not usually as reported from trained meditators. For their part, the Buddhist scholars at the meeting would admit that Buddhist teachings about the mind (the Abhidharma) are not products of "pure" introspective investigation but have also been fundamentally shaped by various classificatory and analytic traditions from Buddhist philosophy. In the end, however, these challenges and admissions would just make the conversation more interesting. In no sense would they negate the basic questions on the table: Could the two traditions work together, and would more be learned about the nature of the mind through the partnership than in its absence?

If better science—a better understanding of the mind—was the initial and official rationale for the scientists' participation, then what about their Buddhist counterparts? Were they at this meeting for the same reasons? For most, at least on some level the answer was yes. By the time they appeared on the stage together, all of the speakers— Buddhist scholars and scientists—had been in conversation for some months. Much of their preliminary work had been focused on shaping their presentations in ways that would maximize the potential for productive discussion afterward. What would be interesting for Buddhists about what the scientists had to say? In the course of exploring this question, a sense of surprised collegiality and shared intellectual energy had begun to emerge. One of the monks, French-born Matthieu Ricard, had been based at the Shechen monastery in Nepal for twenty years. Prior to that time, however, he had studied biochemistry at the Institut Pasteur. His growing involvement now in the neurophysiology of various advanced meditative states (as gleaned in part from data taken from images of his own brain) led him to exclaim about how, after forty years, he had finally returned to science—and to wonder what his old teachers would say![9]

The Buddhist scholars had other motivations, as well, for participating in the meeting, and these became increasingly evident over the course of the two-day conference. Some were motivated by a simple desire to be generous-minded. It was true, they agreed, that they did not need neuroscience (as MIT psychologist Nancy Kanwisher pointed out) to "tell them how to live," but they were happy to help the scientists with their work by answering questions and offering their thoughts. Others believed that collaboration with science was good for Buddhism. "Religions as a whole are prone to ossification and dogmatism," Tibetan Buddhism scholar (and former monk) Alan Wallace told a *Boston Globe* reporter before the conference began. Engaging with modern science, he said, "may really help rescue Buddhism from this tendency."[10] While one result of the meeting might be that some Buddhist claims would be challenged, there was an equal possibility, the Buddhists on stage thought, that science would find some of its presuppositions about human nature challenged. At the very least, the dialogue with science offered the prospect of creating a new pool of evidence for the benefits of meditative practice. Such a result would be useful today because, in the words of Theravada Buddhist monk Ajahn Amaro (who has a degree in psychology and physiology from the University of London), "people believe in the great god of data."

As the meeting progressed, however, more radical agendas on the Buddhist side would begin to emerge that would threaten to destabilize the original vision of Buddhism and science as two investigatory traditions simply swapping questions and sharing insights. It was important to realize, some would say, that in the end Buddhists are interested in investigating the mind for a very different reason than are scientists. In Buddhism, as Alan Wallace said, "the pursuit of knowledge, if it's to go very, very far, is inextricably related to the pursuit of virtue. And the pursuit of virtue is inextricably related to the pursuit of happiness." Put another way, the Buddhists explained, ignorance in their tradition is believed to be the root cause of suffering and wrong action, while knowledge that reflects an accurate grasp of reality is believed to have an ethically transforming effect on the knower. Harvard psychologist Jerome Kagan seized immediately on the incompatibilities between this understanding of knowledge and the usual assumptions of Western science about the relationship between knowledge and ethics. In the Western tradition of science, he noted, "we can have an absolutely amoral scientist discovering a beautiful truth about nature . . . We're using [the word] *knowledge* in different ways." Conference participants and audience members alike were thus invited to consider the possibility that any program to investigate the mind that was forged in the nexus of a full dialogue with Buddhism might ultimately be called upon to consider the ways in which Western science is changed and touched by the knowledge it acquires for itself.

When Mind and Life chairman Adam Engle completed his welcoming remarks, he introduced MIT president Charles Vest, who welcomed the audience on behalf of his university:

Recent scientific advances in study of the brain and mind build on the rapidly accelerating progress in a broad range of disciplines . . . But at the most profound level these studies challenge those of us in the sciences and technologies to go still further afield, to grapple with insights and challenges from the world's great philosophical and spiritual traditions.

That is why this conference is important. It brings together scientists, academics, and Buddhist scholar-practitioners, all distinguished in their own fields, to explore topics of common concern in the spirit of open, honest inquiry that is the essence of the university.

Vest then turned the podium over to Phillip Sharp, director of the McGovern Institute for Brain Research, which cosponsored the conference with Mind and Life. The McGovern Institute was founded in 2000 with the largest single gift ever given to a university (from Patrick J. McGovern and Lore Harp McGovern, both successful entrepreneurs). Its remit was simply to become the world's leading center for cutting-edge integrative neuroscience. Though not trained as a neuroscientist, Sharp was deemed to have the interdisciplinary vision and scientific ambition to realize this audacious goal. In 1993 he shared the Nobel Prize in Physiology or Medicine for the groundbreaking discovery that DNA contains introns (intervening DNA segments that do not code for proteins) and that one function of RNA is to "edit" these out and splice together the remaining exons (meaningful patterns of DNA) to create proteins.

Why had an organization like the McGovern Institute for Brain Research been willing to lend its name—not to speak of the time and energy of some of its scientists—to an event such as this? A critical catalyst here had been Sharp's close colleague Eric Lander, director of the Whitehead Institute/MIT Center for Genome Research (now part of the Broad Institute in Cambridge, Massachusetts). In 2002 Lander had traveled to Dharamsala to spend five days at a Mind and Life meeting between the Dalai Lama and Lander's fellow scientists, at which they discussed the lofty theme, "What Is Matter? What Is Life?" His departure for that meeting had been preceded by a great send-off organized by his staff at the Whitehead Institute, which included twenty Tibetans. The Tibetans gave him a written message to be delivered to the Dalai Lama and told him to "go forward with a clear mind."[11]

He must have done so; at any rate, Lander liked what he saw in Dharamsala. "Science is posing ethical questions today that need to be answered urgently. For me, this conference is really about posing those questions to Buddhism and looking at the reactions," he told a reporter in Dharamsala at that time. "I have a lot of respect for the thoughtful dialogue that happened. No one was trying to convince the other. They were trying to open perspectives, which can always do with a bit of opening."[12] Lander's experience served as the starting point for his pitch to the McGovern Institute to consider cosponsoring a public meeting that some elite universities and scientific institutions might have considered too risky to their image. Scientists and others at the McGovern Institute listened to him and agreed to do it. In the end, they could agree to do it, as Lander cheerfully explained a few weeks before the conference, because both MIT and the McGovern Institute were secure enough in their scientific reputations not to fear pushing the envelope a bit.

On stage now, it was Phillip Sharp's job to introduce the Dalai Lama himself. He did so with the following words:

He is the fourteenth Dalai Lama, leader of Tibetan Buddhism and head of the Tibetan government in exile. He was born of very humble origins and was selected to be the Dalai Lama at the age of two. His Holiness has an advanced degree in Buddhist philosophy and has been educated by participating on the world's stage for over forty years. He is truly an international scholar and leader. One recognition of the importance of his leadership was the awarding of the Nobel Peace Prize [to him] in 1989.

I had the pleasure yesterday of attending a press conference with His Holiness. Two attributes stood out as I listened to his responses to questions. The first was his openness to insights learned through scientific inquiry. I believe this reflects a very deep personal interest in him, since His Holiness secondly said something that's very important for MIT, that if he were not a monk, he would have liked to have been an engineer.

The audience laughed appreciatively. Sharp concluded his remarks, and there was an expectant pause. It was finally the Dalai Lama's turn to rise and address the audience. On some level, probably everyone in the auditorium that day—audience members as well as the scientists and Buddhist scholars on the stage—had been waiting above all to hear him speak. This was an academic conference, but it was also—let us admit it—an opportunity for all those present to have some sort of encounter with one of the best-loved and most intriguing spiritual leaders of our time.

It is worth noting that, had a meeting of this sort with the Dalai Lama been organized a mere twenty years earlier, it would not have had nearly the same cultural and emotional valence. Though Tibetan Buddhism had been slowly winning a modest base of American followers since the 1960s (a consequence of lamas coming to this country in the wake of the invasion of their country by the Chinese),[13] Buddhism had nevertheless remained an obscure tradition for most Americans right into the 1980s—and the Dalai Lama an equally obscure figure. As the *Boston Globe* reported, when the Dalai Lama came to the United States for the first time in 1978 and his followers "called TV programs to ask if they cared to interview the Dalai Lama, frequently the response was, 'What did you say her last name was?'"[14]

The emergence of the Dalai Lama as a famous spiritual teacher in the Western world owes much to the advocacy and publicity work of one of his most devoted followers, Robert Thurman, founder of the Tibet House cultural center in New York and professor of Buddhist studies at Columbia University.[15] It was Thurman who successfully nominated the Dalai Lama for the Nobel Peace Prize in 1989, recognizing his nonviolent efforts to work with China toward a solution to the "Tibet question." That same year, a horrified world had watched televised images of the Chinese government using tanks to suppress its own students, who were peacefully protesting in Tiananmen Square. The Dalai Lama's pacifist approach seemed all the more impressive through the contrast, and the message of international disapproval of China's government that was conveyed through awarding the Tibetan leader such a prize was unambiguous.

After winning the 1989 Nobel Peace Prize, the Dalai Lama traveled ever more frequently to the West, and his smiling face and charismatic presence became intricately associated with a long-standing romantic view of Tibet as a real-life Shangri-la, untouched by the corrupting influences of modern society. Many in the West began to see Tibet as a repository of unique spiritual insight that just might be in a position to rescue a morally bankrupt and spiritually lost world from itself.[16]

The West's embracing of the Dalai Lama as an emissary from Shangri-la is not without irony, given that the better informed of his followers realize that he is actually at the forefront of a "Buddhist modernization" movement. His ongoing dialogue with science over the years is at the heart of his efforts in this direction. At the conference at MIT, he noted that "one of the facts of our modern society is that all of humanity has faith and confidence in science, as well as an admiration for science," and he implicitly included himself among its admirers. In his autobiography, he writes at length of his personal fascination with science and technology—how, as a boy being groomed to take up his post as Dalai Lama in Tibet, he liked nothing better than to tinker with Western gadgets that had found their way into his homeland, from watches to an old cinema projector (which he got working without recourse to a manual). Thupten Jinpa, who translated for the Dalai Lama at the MIT meeting, has suggested that the Dalai Lama's recognition of the social benefits of science and technology "may have come during his state visits to China in 1955 and to India in 1956. The impact of the powerful industries and modern telecommunication and transport systems on the young Dalai Lama's mind [should not] be underestimated."[17]

At the same time that the West began to embrace the Dalai Lama as the human face of an ancient spiritual tradition, the Dalai Lama himself, Thupten Jinpa tells us, began speaking in public, especially at major academic monastic colleges, about the need to introduce studies of modern science and Western philosophy into the monastic curriculum. "If science proves facts that conflict with Buddhist understanding," the Dalai Lama often said, "Buddhism must change accordingly. We should always adopt a view that accords with the facts."[18] Thupten Jinpa notes further that "the Dalai Lama does not see the introduction of modern science within the classical curriculum as something radical. Rather he sees this more as a matter of updating the curriculum. He argues that the study of physics updates the student's understanding of the nature of the physical universe, [and similarly sees] cosmology as updating classical Buddhist cosmology, biology as [updating] the study of life and consciousness, and psychology as updating the study of classical Abhidharma psychology and phenomenology."[19]

It was not, however, strictly his personal admiration for science, nor his modernizing ambitions for Tibetan monastic culture, that had brought the Dalai Lama to MIT. He was also there because he believed that, as a team, Western science and Buddhism (and other ancient Asian spiritual traditions, he was quick to insist) could contribute more to human welfare than each could on its own. In what way was this the case? As he now stood and addressed the audience in Kresge Auditorium that morning, he tried to explain: "Everyone strives for material comfort, but there is inadequate attention paid to inner values. One of my commitments—and not just mine alone—is to try to promote human values in ways that might lead to a happier world and a more compassionate world." What was the best way, though, to promote human values in the modern world? He went on:

Not through prayer, not through religious teaching, but through awareness. What I have learned in the past several years, in the course of meetings with scientists, is that the brain cannot develop properly and people cannot be healthy in the absence of human affection. I see in such scientific findings some kind of backing for the promoting of human values. In order to have a healthy body, you must have a happy mind. . . So I now have a few more reasons for urging people to practice the cultivation of values: developmental reasons, health reasons, peace of mind reasons. All suggest the combination of brain and heart is something very crucial. In this context, meetings between science and older traditions like Buddhism can be very useful.

The Dalai Lama stressed to the audience, "I'm not making an effort to propagate Buddhism or to try to demonstrate to other people that it is something very special. I don't think that way." There were doubtless many spiritual traditions, he said—Hindu, Christian, Jewish, Sufi—that could equally partner with science in the service of the same kind of end. Indeed, he added, "in some cases I feel that with Buddhists, particularly ones like myself without much experience, there's a lot of blah, blah, blah." The audience laughed. "Bringing in experienced people from a wide range of traditions could therefore be very worthwhile" for the research effort. At the same time, introducing a multifaith dimension to the effort, he said, could help contribute to a larger goal of promoting "religious harmony."

That said, there was just one way in which he did hope that Tibetan Buddhism, specifically, might benefit from being involved in a public dialogue with scientists. "Some of our Chinese brothers and sisters consider Tibetan traditions to be very backward," he said in closing. The fact that so many prominent Western scientists find those traditions both rich and relevant to their own work could help change such perceptions, he explained. In this way it could help persuade the Chinese that Tibetan culture is worth preserving, and contribute to the ongoing political effort to win back for Tibet some measure of cultural autonomy. "I want to show them," he declared firmly as he ended his remarks, "that we are not so backward."

It was now time for Arthur Zajonc and me to rise and begin our job as moderators of the conference. Both of us had been involved with the Mind and Life Institute for some years and had participated in one or more of the private meetings in Dharamsala, and we believed in the integrity and value of the dialogue process. We are neither neuroscientists nor Buddhist scholars. Arthur is a physicist with strong philosophical interests and a track record of engagement with pedagogical innovation. I am a historian of science with a special interest in the contemporary mind and brain sciences and what they tell us— and also perhaps don't tell us—about the nature of our humanness. Through previous projects, I had also developed a strong interest in interdisciplinary exchanges between the natural sciences and the humanities: what they can achieve, how to enable them, ways in which they can go wrong. I hoped that my experience in this area would serve me in good stead over the next two days.

As we approached the podium, we also both hoped that our status as official outsiders to the two traditions in dialogue during this meeting would be more useful than not. Because we did not claim to be experts, we had license to ask the kinds of questions of clarification that members of the audience might wish they could ask. With no particular stake in any specific debate, our job was simply to keep the dialogue flowing as coherently as possible, and to briefly halt the action when necessary to sharpen, gloss, or summarize a point that might otherwise have been obscured. As editors of this volume, which attempts to capture both the content and the spirit of the two-day meeting at MIT, we will continue to serve in that same role for our readers.

EVAN THOMPSON

Neurophenomenology and Francisco Varela

CHAPTER TWO

Francisco Varela was a neurobiologist who worked on the biology of cognition; he was also a practitioner of Buddhist meditation, a student of Buddhist philosophy, and a cofounder of the Mind and Life Institute. He was a pioneer not only in neuroscience, immunology, theoretical biology, and cognitive science, but also in the exchange between Western science and Buddhism.[1] During the last decade of his life, Varela made groundbreaking experimental and theoretical contributions to our understanding of the large-scale, dynamic brain processes involved in perception and consciousness.[2] Yet he was never content to investigate simply the neural correlates of mind. Varela wanted to understand the nature of experience itself. In his view, there could be no comprehensive science of the mind without understanding subjective experience, especially the subjective experience of one's own mental processes as they are lived in the first person.

Varela maintained, furthermore, that scientific understanding of subjective experience requires linking biobehavioral investigations of the mind to rigorous and precise phenomenological investigations. He believed that Buddhism, because of its long-standing traditions of disciplined, contemplative study of the mind and critical philosophical analysis, has deep and extensive contributions to make to the scientific investigation of the mind. Thus Varela's vision was not that Buddhist contemplatives could become new subjects (or objects) for experimental research on the neural correlates of mental states, but rather that adept contemplative phenomenologists could become a new kind of scientific collaborator or partner in investigating the mind.

More than one hundred years ago, William James, in his *Principles of Psychology*, wrote that in the study of subjective mental phenomena, "Introspective Observation is what we have to rely on first and foremost and always."[3] Psychology, as James presented it, is the study of subjective mental phenomena, plus their relations to their objects, to brain states, and to the environment. Whereas physiological psychology studies the relation of mind and brain, as well as the naturally evolved "mutual fit" of mental faculties and the environment, introspection studies the subjective mental states themselves. Yet what exactly is introspection? James continued: "The word introspection need hardly be defined—it means, of course, the looking into our own minds and reporting what we there discover. *Everyone agrees that we there discover states of consciousness.*"[4]

This passage is often quoted, but less often remarked is that James hardly thought introspection was an easy or infallible guide to subjective mental life. Later in his book, when discussing sensed moments of transition in the subjective stream of thought and feeling, he wrote: "Let anyone try to cut a thought across in the middle and get a look at its section, and he will see how difficult the introspective observation of the transitive tracts is . . . The attempt at introspective analysis in these cases is in fact like seizing a spinning top to catch its motion, or trying to turn up the gas quickly enough to see how the darkness looks."[5]

James clearly did not think that we know the nature and full range of thought and feeling simply because we are able to look into our own minds. In 1904 James heard the Theravada Buddhist renunciate Anagarika Dharmapala lecture at Harvard on the Buddhist conception of mind. According to the Buddhist view, he learned, there is no single, permanent, enduring self underlying the stream of mental and physical events. Afterward, James rose and proclaimed to the audience, "This is the psychology everybody will be studying twenty-five years from now." By this he apparently meant not so much Buddhist psychology per se, but rather a psychology of the full developmental range of human consciousness, pursued with the kind of phenomenological precision exemplified by Buddhism.[6]

James's prediction, of course, was too optimistic. The words of another psychologist, James McKeen Cattell, also from 1904, indicate the path that much of psychology would take in the years to come: "It is usually no more necessary for the subject in a psychology experiment to be a psychologist than it is for the vivisected frog to be a physiologist."[7] The strategy psychology pursued was to objectify the mind as much as possible, either as behavioral performance, physiological response, or nonconscious information processing. *Consciousness* became a taboo term, introspection was rejected as a method for investigating the mind, and it was no longer necessary for the psychologist to have any disciplined first-person expertise in the investigation of mental life. Although there were notable exceptions to this trend, such as Gestalt psychology and phenomenological psychology, this "taboo of subjectivity" influenced the scientific study of the mind for decades.[8]

It has taken us more than a full century, not a quarter of one, to find our way back to James's vision of a science of mental life that integrates experimental psychology, brain science, and phenomenology. In recent years, a growing number of cognitive scientists have come to accept that there cannot be a complete science of the mind without an understanding of subjectivity and consciousness, and that cognitive science will accordingly need to make systematic use of introspective "first-person" reports about subjective experience.[9] As the cognitive neuroscientist Chris Frith recently stated: "A major programme for 21st century science will be to discover how an experience can be translated into a report, thus enabling our experiences to be shared."[10]

This renewed appreciation of subjective experience raises the question of how to obtain precise phenomenological data. Varela was especially concerned with this question in his research on the neurodynamics of mental states. His proposal was that cognitive neuroscience needs to incorporate what he called first-person methods of exploring experience.[11] First-person methods increase an individual's sensitivity to his or her own experience through the systematic training of attention and self-regulation of emotion. First-person methods are important for cognitive neuroscience for several reasons, Varela believed. First, they help subjects gain access to aspects of their experience that would otherwise remain unnoticed, such as their transient affective state or quality of attention. Second, the refined first-person reports subjects produce can help the experimenter to understand physiological processes that would otherwise remain opaque, such as the variability in brain dynamics as seen in neuroimaging experiments. Varela called this approach "neurophenomenology."[12] He demonstrated its fruitfulness in one of his last experimental studies, in which first-person methods were used to reveal important phenomenological differences in the subjective quality of attention during visual perception, and these differences were shown to be correlated with distinct frequency and phase-synchrony patterns in the large-scale dynamics of brain activity on a millisecond time-scale.[13]

There is another reason Varela believed first-person methods to be important. Individuals who can generate specific sorts of mental states and report on those states with a high degree of phenomenological precision provide a route into studying the causal efficacy of mental processes, considered neurodynamically as global or large-scale processes that can modify local neural and somatic events. Varela believed that reintroducing the causal efficacy of the mental in this way was theoretically and experimentally more fruitful than the standard neural-correlates framework, and he developed these ideas in his pioneering research on the neurodynamics of epilepsy and strategies for the first-person cognitive control of epileptic seizures.[14]

It is worth reconsidering, from this vantage point of first-person methods, why psychology rejected introspection long ago. According to the standard history, introspection was given a fair try but failed. It failed allegedly because the two rival schools of introspectionist psychology were unable to agree whether there was such a thing as imageless thought. James had already observed, however, that the form of introspection practiced by these schools was stilted and tedious, because it focused on the sensations caused by tedious and impoverished sensory stimuli.[15] It is not surprising that introspection of this sort turned out to be so unilluminating, as Gestalt psychologists and phenomenologists also later pointed out.[16] Furthermore, the textbook history neglects to mention that the rival schools did agree with each other at the descriptive level of introspective phenomenology; their disagreement was at the level of theoretical interpretation. One lesson to be learned from this debate, therefore, is not that introspection is a useless method for obtaining descriptive data about subjective experience, but that psychology needs to discriminate carefully between the description of subjective phenomena and causal-explanatory theorizing.[17] A similar lesson should be drawn from the famous studies of Nisbett and Wilson in 1977: they observed that subjects often said their behavior was caused by mental events when it was really the result of external manipulation.[18] Yet these inaccurate subjective reports were causal-explanatory in form, not purely descriptive and phenomenological. Again the lesson to be learned is that subjects should be coached to pay strict attention to their felt cognitive processes and to avoid causal-explanatory conjectures.[19]

Yet how is such attention to be cultivated? Varela saw first-person methods as concerned with precisely this question, and he viewed Buddhist practices of contemplative mental discipline as exemplary because of their pragmatic refinement and theoretical sophistication. Whereas James described introspection as simply "the looking into our own minds and reporting what we there discover," Buddhism speaks of sustained voluntary attention to one's own mental processes.

Buddhist phenomenology distinguishes between attentional stability and instability due to mental excitation, and between attentional vividness and dullness due to mental laxity. Buddhist phenomenology also discusses the metacognitive monitoring of these qualities of attention, and Buddhist epistemology discusses the degree to which a state of mental cognition ascertains or fails to ascertain its object, under various conditions.[20] According to this perspective, if the stream of thought and feeling is limpid, rather than turbulent and murky, then introspection in James's sense will be much richer in its discoveries and reports.

I already noted that Varela's vision was not that Buddhist contemplatives could become new experimental subjects for research on the neural correlates of consciousness, but rather that they could become a new kind of scientific collaborator or partner. Cognitive science has so far explored only one small area of the human mind—the one accessible to phenomenologically naive subjects reporting to phenomenologically naive cognitive scientists. The encounter between Buddhism and cognitive science raises another prospect—that of subjects with a high degree of phenomenological expertise reporting to phenomenologically informed cognitive scientists. Varela's vision, in its boldest and most provocative form, was that future cognitive neuroscientists would be trained in contemplative phenomenology as well as brain-imaging techniques and mathematical modeling; at the same time, contemplative phenomenologists would be knowledgeable in neuroscience and experimental psychology. The two perspectives would mutually constrain and enrich each other, and would hybridize into the rich science of mental life James originally envisioned. Francisco Varela's hope, I believe, was that volumes such as this one could be a first step on this journey.

II

ATTENTION
AND
COGNITIVE
CONTROL

JONATHAN COHEN

Understandings of Attention and Cognitive Control from Cognitive Neuroscience

The "Investigating the Mind" conference at MIT took three topics—attention, imagery, and emotion—as its points of focus in the dialogue between Western cognitive neuroscience and Buddhism. There was a lot of discussion among organizers of the conference as to which of the three topics should go first. Each was important and seemed to generate a great amount of interest and enthusiasm. In the end the choice was largely arbitrary. The rationale—such as it was—for beginning with attention and cognitive control was that these phenomena play a central role in Buddhist practice and philosophy and, of course, the topic is of great interest in modern psychology.

I would now like to outline some of the things that we have learned about attention using scientific methodology and, maybe more important, some of the limitations in what we have learned. I hope these perspectives from cognitive neuroscience will prove to complement the perspectives derived from Buddhist approaches and can then be further explored. I begin with some definitions, because if we are going to have a dialogue between different cultures that are accustomed to using different languages, it is important that each side does its best to define its terms. On the scientific side, it has been a problem even getting *scientists* to agree about what is meant by attention and cognitive control. The definitions that I'm going to put forward in these remarks are therefore just a starting point for discussion and should not be taken too rigidly. Nevertheless I do think they capture much of the current consensus of scientific thinking about attention and cognitive control.

By "attention" we typically mean the capacity to process selectively information that is available to us. This is captured in the famous quote by William James: "Every one knows what attention is. It is the taking possession by the mind, in clear and vivid form, of one out of what seem several simultaneously possible objects or trains of thought. Focalization, concentration, of consciousness are of its essence. It implies withdrawal from some things in order to deal effectively with others."[1]

The focus can be on information that is sensory, it can consist of bodily feelings, or it can consist of thoughts, memories, or even actions. Much of my concern is with the relationship of attention to control, but insofar as it is possible to talk about cognitive control as something different than attention, what we mean is the capacity to guide thought and behavior in accord with intention. "Cognitive control" refers to an internal directing of behavior, often most evident when we have to override a habitual or reflexive response. My favorite example is the choice not to scratch a mosquito bite. It's compelling, the urge to scratch a mosquito bite. Often, if we're distracted, we will find ourselves scratching. Yet we have the capability not to scratch. The purpose of control is to restrain certain behaviors in favor of pursuing other, more interesting strategies and goals.

One of the reasons that attentional mechanisms exist in the brain, or in the mind, is that there is more information in the environment than our minds can apprehend at any one time. In the laboratory we often use an experiment for "change blindness," which illustrates this limitation in our ability to process information and underscores why attention is so important.[2] The experiment involves flashing at subjects a set of pictures that change in some unspecified way. The goal is to see how quickly the subject can detect what is changing. In one typical example, a reflection on the water in a pair of otherwise identical photographs comes in and out of view. Once you see the difference between the images, it is almost impossible not to see it, and yet the change is very hard to notice at first, when the pictures are quickly alternating.

The change-blindness experiment illustrates just how focused our attention can be. We refer to this as the limited capacity of attention. It's difficult for people to attend to many sources of information at once or even to many parts of the same source of information. Similarly, it's difficult to perform many controlled, demanding tasks at once. For example, when we first learn to ride a bike or drive a car, we don't want somebody talking to us while we do it. After we have gotten better at it perhaps it's okay to have a conversation at the same time, but when we are first learning, we need to focus our attention. It's hard to do two things at once.

Another insight that has come out of research in psychology is that there is a continuum in the need for attention control.[3] As just noted, when we are first learning to drive a car we must give the task a lot of attention, but over time, as we gain experience and practice, the same task requires less attention. Once we have enough experience, we can drive a car almost without thinking about it. This fact in turn raises one of the central questions of psychological research in this area: How are attention and control related to each other? There are two answers: they are the same, and they are different.

First I want to describe what they have in common. Those who think of attention and control as the same thing take the view that attention is essentially what control does. Control operates by representing the goal of a behavior: what we are trying to accomplish. It then oversees the process of performing the particular task to achieve the goal by selecting appropriate stimuli and the actions that correspond to those stimuli. It selects the right things to process and decides what we want to do with them. The observable effects of this interaction are what we call attention.

How can we study this in the laboratory? I offered one example above, but there are many others. For example, we can observe subjects performing a task that engages spatial attention—the ability to locate objects in a particular part of space. The task seems simple at first: we show the subjects a group of short lines on a screen, one of which is horizontal while all the rest are slanted, and we ask them to locate the horizontal line. For most people, the horizontal line seems to pop right out of the group, and in fact this is commonly referred to as the "pop-out effect." Similarly, if we ask subjects to locate a single short red line within a group of short green lines, that line also seems to pop right out. It's almost as if the task did not require attention. However, if we present subjects with an array of both horizontal and diagonal short lines, the horizontal lines all green but one, the diagonal lines both red and green, and tell them to look for the line that is horizontal and red, that task is much harder. The display on the screen is more or less the same, but subjects find that they have to scan the options sequentially.[4] Their attention is engaged, and it turns out that, in this instance, they have to control that attention; they must actively seek until they actually find the target.

Tasks like these give us an opportunity to test which circumstances engage attention and which ones don't. We can measure, for example, the relationship between how long it takes to find a target and the number of distracters there are. In other words, such tasks offer a way of measuring demands on attention. Anne Treisman, who participated in the dialogue at MIT, has pioneered the research in this area.[5]

In addition to asking subjects to focus their attention on the location of one object among many, we can also direct them to focus on picking out particular features of a single object. The Stroop test, named for the researcher who first described it more than seventy years ago, is a test in which the words for colors are written in colors that conflict with the words' meanings (the word *green*, for example, is printed in red letters).[6] This test has been used more than any other to study attention in the psychology laboratory.[7] Among the many findings is that people are much slower to name the color shown when the meaning of the word contradicts the color of the letters. If the word *green* were printed in green, then the task would be much easier. The Stroop test illustrates our ability to attend to one dimension of a stimulus, and also the difficulty we sometimes have in making our attention complete—in processing exclusively what we want to process without interference from other sources of information.

The test should be equally effective in a cross-cultural context, and we tried a variation of the Stroop test using Tibetan words for colors, written in colors that conflicted with the words' meanings (the Tibetan word for "green" was printed in red, for example). When asked to name just the color shown and to ignore the word itself, the Tibetan subjects we tested—including, informally, the Dalai Lama himself—found it difficult to ignore the word's meaning.

A particularly interesting aspect of attention revealed by this and similar tests is the observation that when attempts are made to focus attention in this way (that is, to attend to the color and ignore the word), it appears that specific parts of the brain are actively engaged. The area involved includes the prefrontal cortex, a part of the brain lying just behind the forehead that has consistently been associated with higher-level functions that rely on cognitive control.[8]

We have observed this in many different contexts, not only in the Stroop test and others similar to it but also when attention or control is needed to override emotions.[9] Studies have been done in which subjects are presented with moral dilemmas involving a conflict between emotion and rational thought or cognition. In one example, a subject is asked to imagine him or herself in a town attacked by enemy soldiers. The townspeople, including the subject, all decide to hide. Everybody has to be quiet; if the soldiers find them, they will kill everyone. Suddenly a baby begins to cry. What should the subject do? Should he or she—or the mother—cover the baby and risk suffocating it in order to save all the townspeople?

We have found that the subjects who respond emotionally to this moral challenge—those who say they could not risk the baby's life—

show activity in areas of the brain that are associated with emotion. In contrast, the subjects who decide that risking the baby's life, however horrible, is acceptable because it will likely save more lives show greater activity in the prefrontal cortex.[10] We believe that this brain activity is related to the effort of overcoming emotion. In other words, the same region of the brain that is active in focusing attention is also active in overriding and controlling the emotional response that might otherwise lead to a different kind of behavior.

We see the same kind of emotional and control processes engaged in economic decision making. In one experiment, a man is given a hundred dollars and is told that he must share it with a partner, but that it is his job to decide how to split it up. He decides to offer his partner a penny and keep $99.99 for himself. The partner (the true subject of this study) may very naturally be offended and may even reject the offer in anger. When we have done brain scans of people who are presented with this situation and reject the offer, we find that the areas of their brain related to emotion are activated.[11] Other subjects, however, decide that a penny is better than nothing and accept the offer; these people show greater activity in their prefrontal cortex. One part of the mind, presumably associated with control, can overcome the emotional response of perceived injury and lead to what some may argue is more rational behavior (after all, a penny is better than nothing).

These observations suggest that control and attention are very closely related. Control leads to the focusing of attention on sensory events or actions that lead, in turn, to a particular behavior. At the same time, other observations suggest that the two phenomena are different: that, specifically, internal control reflects one source of attention—a voluntary sort—but that other sorts of attention work differently. For example, a sudden stimulus can capture attention without any voluntary desire to attend to that stimulus. This suggests that attention might be considered more generally, then, to be the selective effect of whatever is currently guiding thought. In some instances, that might be a goal or intention that comes from internal control; in others it might be a stimulus, a memory, or a particularly powerful emotion that might not be under internal control. Thus there may indeed be a difference between attention in general and internal control. Buddhists and cognitive scientists share an interest in this possibility.

So, against this background, what are the questions that appear to be most fruitful for cross-cultural dialogue, from the point of view of cognitive neuroscience?

The first and perhaps most interesting question has already been raised: are attention and control unitary mechanisms? In other words, is there a single mechanism of attention? Is the same mechanism that is used to pay attention to the color of a stimulus, for example, also used to find the location of a stimulus, or to control an emotion? Much psychological research suggests the mechanisms may be different, which raises the possibility that there could be a family of mechanisms that share some things in common but are different in other ways.

If there are differences between various forms of attention and control, how can we describe them more precisely? Of these different forms, which ones are most relevant to Buddhist practice? Which will be most illuminated in the course of discussions with Buddhist practitioners?

If there are indeed many forms of attention, we could also ask how focused or broad each one is. To study this, subjects might be presented with a display of letters of different sizes—such as a large S shape made up of small H's—and be asked to identify the small letters or the large ones, or to say what words the letters combine to make. Subjects could be asked to look at specific features that are spatially localized, for which they may use single sensory channels, and they could be asked to distribute their attention spatially over the whole scene to get the gist of it. We could then see if the same mechanism that is involved in focused attention is also involved in a more panoramic form of attention. Again, is there one mechanism underlying attention or are there several?

Another question came out of our previous discussions with Buddhist practitioners: What are the timing characteristics of human attention? Measured in the laboratory and using normal subjects, it is commonly found that a percept needs 50 to 100 milliseconds of stability to command attention. Yet discussions with our Buddhist colleagues suggest that a highly trained mind may be able to attend to one event per millisecond, which represents a much more compressed time scale.

We are also interested in engaging in a dialogue with our Buddhist colleagues about the nature of selective versus sustained attention. In initial explorations of attention, psychologists were very interested in the enduring capability of attention: how long people can remain vigilant. Over the past ten or twenty years, much of the focus has shifted to studies of the selective aspects of attention, and we currently know less than we might about the mind's ability to sustain attention; here, we may be able to learn a lot from Buddhist practitioners.

From preliminary conversations with our Buddhist (primarily Tibetan Buddhist) colleagues, it seems that the two traditions—Western cognitive neuroscience and Buddhism—think of the relationship between attention and effort differently. We scientists tend to think of attention as effortful and to believe that it is difficult to maintain a selective or enduring focus of attention over a long period of time. In Buddhist practice it appears that, at least after initial training, focusing attention is an effortless and almost relaxing process. If true, this is of great interest to us.

Finally, perhaps the most important question we have concerns how capabilities relating to attention and control can be cultivated, can be learned. In the tradition I represent, researchers have spent much time studying how, when one learns a skill, reliance on attention is reduced. However, very little research has been done on the extent to which one can learn to *control* attention. In contrast, such training of the attention is an essential feature of Buddhist practice.

I will close by just mentioning two phenomena related to attention and cognitive control that have long been recognized in Western science but have remained on the fringes of study: placebo effects and hypnosis. In Western behavioral science we think of these phenomena as products of heightened expectation, or selective attention, which can lead to a change in a person's experience, including a bodily change. If a doctor tells a person that a medicine will help him and he believes it, then even a sugar pill—a placebo—may be able to improve his health. Similarly with hypnosis: focused attention can lead to unusual abilities and experiences.

In both these cases, though, the ability to focus attention or control in unusual ways is triggered by an external force: the authority of the doctor or the hypnotist. It would be interesting to explore how these kinds of experiences compare with the types of heightened control over bodily experience and behavior that Buddhists suggest can be achieved through internal direction.

B. ALAN WALLACE

Buddhist Training in Enhanced Attention Skills

I wish to present a Buddhist perspective on ways of training the attention, the nature of attention, and the plasticity of attention. First, to relate this perspective to Western psychology, let us turn again to the American pioneer of psychology, William James, who set forth a threefold strategy for studying the mind. The discipline, he proposed, should include three avenues for studying mental states and activity: (1) indirectly, by way of their behavioral correlates; (2) indirectly, by way of their neural correlates; and (3) directly, by way of the introspective examination of subjective mental phenomena themselves. Among these approaches, he declared, "Introspective observation is what we have to rely on first and foremost and always."[1]

James wrote brilliantly about attention generally, and specifically about what he called sustained voluntary attention. He was a broad-ranging thinker concerned with a wide variety of topics, including philosophy and education. In this context, he addressed the relevance of attention to many human endeavors. In regard to education, for example, he commented: "The faculty of voluntarily bringing back a wandering attention, over and over again, is the very root of judgment, character and will. An education which should improve this faculty would be the education par excellence. But it is easier to define this ideal than to give practical instructions for bringing it about."[2]

James thought that the control of attention was of paramount importance for making ethical decisions and determining what we actually experience in the world. "For the moment," he declared, "what we attend to is reality."[3] While he viewed the control of attention to be of the highest importance, he was not optimistic about the possibility of training to help achieve this goal: "The possession of such a steady faculty of attention is unquestionably a great boon. Those who have it can work more rapidly, and with less nervous wear and tear. I am inclined to think that no one who is without it naturally can by any amount of drill or discipline attain it in a very high degree. Its amount is probably a fixed characteristic of the individual."[4]

Since the time of William James, we have seen tremendous progress in the behavioral sciences and in neuroscience. But in terms of the introspective study of the mind, the cognitive sciences have stayed more or less at a standstill. In fact, in light of the growing prevalence of attention disorders, the attention skills of modern society actually seem to be advancing to the rear.

Buddhism, unlike Western science, has always had a central interest in the nature of the mind. Centuries before the time of the Buddha, who lived 2,500 years ago, extraordinary advances had already been made in terms of gaining cognitive control of attention, and by his own account the Buddha was a beneficiary of this earlier tradition of training the attention. After applying himself to such training under the guidance of two contemplative adepts, he incorporated it into his teachings on the path to liberation, and such training has remained a central feature of Buddhist contemplative practice ever since.

Buddhist practice is not confined to training the attention, of course. The Buddhist study of the mind exists in a much broader context. The foundation of Buddhist practice is ethics, without which there can be no viable spiritual practice at all. According to Buddhism, this is a universal truth. It is not confined to Buddhism. It is not a sectarian issue. It is just the way things are. But it is not simply a dogmatic assertion. An ethical way of life—a way of life that is oriented toward not injuring others and to being of service where one can—is a life based on empathy, compassion, and altruism, and pragmatically, such a life turns out to be a foundation for achieving mental health and balance. Achieving such balance requires the cultivation of attentional and emotional balance as well as cognitive balance. Cognitive balance consists of clearly seeing what is presented to our senses, without superimposing things that are not there.

Ethics and the exceptional mental health embodied in a balanced mind form the basis for the cultivation of contemplative insight, the cutting edge of Buddhist practice that is designed to heal the mind irreversibly of its afflictions. The cultivation of such insight involves the experiential investigation of all manner of phenomena. The primary emphasis is on the examination of subjective mental states, but Buddhist inquiry also includes the study of objective physical phenomena, and the relationship between subjective and objective, inner and outer phenomena.

In any interdisciplinary and cross-cultural discussion of the mind, including attention, it is important to ensure that miscommunication does not arise in the use of terminology. Obviously, Tibetans do not speak English as their native language, nor did their Buddhist predecessors in India. The Sanskrit term that I am translating as attention is *manasikāra*. In Buddhist psychology, this is defined as a distinct mental factor having the specific function of directing awareness and other concomitant mental processes to an object, enabling one to apprehend the nature of that object.[5] In Buddhist understanding, there may be multiple simultaneous mental processes that work together and are focused on the same object. For example, as I look at an object I may do so with admiration, desire, or expectation. In each instance a number of mental factors may arise simultaneously, and attention focuses all of them on the same object.

Indian contemplatives even before the time of the Buddha were concerned with the nature and potential of attention, and one of their first discoveries was that normal, untrained attention is impaired. For centuries contemplatives throughout the world have found that it is very difficult to sustain attention voluntarily with a high degree of clarity. Shantideva, one of the most renowned of Indian Buddhist sages, lived in the seventh century and studied and taught at the great monastic university of Nalanda. This was an extraordinary institution of higher learning, with a student body of 10,000 and an eleven-story main library. Located in the north of India, it was one of the principal centers of learning for the whole of Asia, and many of the greatest Buddhist pundits studied and taught there. In his classic treatise, *A Guide to the Bodhisattva Way of Life*, Shantideva commented on one of the consequences of impaired attention: "One should stabilize the mind in meditative concentration, for a person's whose mind is distracted lives between the fangs of mental afflictions."[6]

What Shantideva meant here was that insofar as the mind is prone to excitation, turbulence, and distraction, it is out of control. This clearly implies that, from a Buddhist perspective, attention and cognitive control are not the same. To the extent that attention is out of control, the mind is vulnerable to mental afflictions such as anger, craving, envy, and myriad other mental tendencies that can disrupt its equilibrium, resulting in a great deal of unnecessary suffering. In short, when the mind is distracted, the "psychological immune system" is impaired, making one prone to inner sources of unhappiness.

At roughly the time of the decline of Buddhism in India, Tibetans began establishing their own monastic universities, inspired by Nalanda and other such institutions. The fifteenth-century Tibetan scholar and contemplative Tsongkhapa, who studied extensively in the Tibetan schools, wrote a definitive presentation on the ways of training the attention in which he illustrated its relevance for studying the mind and all other types of phenomena: "In order to examine a wall tapestry in a dark room, if you illuminate it with a radiant, steady lamp, you can vividly examine the images in the tapestry. But if the lamp is either dim, or, even if it is bright, flickers due to wind, your observation will be impaired. Likewise, in order to fathom the nature of any phenomenon, with penetrating intelligence supported by unwavering, sustained, voluntary attention, you can clearly observe the real nature of the phenomenon under investigation."[7]

Buddhism has not developed a marvelous array of technologies like that produced by Western science in the past 400 years, but it has devised methods for developing the faculty of introspection, which provides, after all, our sole access to the direct observation of mental phenomena. Attention training is a crucial element in the Buddhist meditative cultivation of the mind. Such attention training has specific goals, of which the first is relaxation. One proceeds in this practice with a sense of ease; it must not be intensely, ambitiously bound up with hopes and desires. One can certainly exert too much effort. On the basis of relaxation, one cultivates stability, involving coherence and continuity of attention to one's chosen object. But it is not enough for attention to be merely stable. It must also be imbued with a sense of clarity, vividness, and high resolution.

To develop these qualities of attention—stability and vividness—which are useful in every conscious human endeavor, including the first-person investigation of the mind, two faculties are employed. The first of these is mindfulness, which is defined in this tradition as the ability to sustain voluntary attention continuously on a familiar object, without forgetfulness or distraction.[8] The Sanskrit term, translated as mindfulness *(smṛti)*, also means recollection. This suggests a parallel with William James's comment, "What is called sustained voluntary attention is a repetition of successive efforts which bring back the topic to the mind."[9] According to Buddhism, mindfulness is a sequence of pulses of cognition, of remembering to remember.

In the development of attention skills, the employment of mindfulness alone is not enough. If you are attending to something mindfully, how do you know whether your mind has unconsciously "exploded" out into sensory distractions or wandering thoughts, or "imploded" into laxity, dullness, or sleepiness? To recognize such attentional imbalances as soon as they arise, you must develop and apply a kind of meta-attention *(samprajanya)*, which has the function of monitoring the quality of attention. So mindfulness and meta-attention are the two faculties to be developed in the cultivation of attentional stability and vividness.

In the Buddhist understanding, attention in a single moment is said to be highly selective. Whether it is voluntary or involuntary, a single moment of attention is focused on only one of the five physical fields of sensory perception or on the field of mental phenomena, which is considered the sixth domain of immediate experience. For instance, in a single moment one may observe visual phenomena, or mental phenomena—such as emotions, thoughts, and so forth—but not both.

There are signs that the quality of attention is being enhanced. At the beginning of the training, it requires a considerable degree of effort. (If all you want to do is arouse a relaxation response, a more direct method might be to sit back in a Jacuzzi.) As James declared, voluntarily bringing back one's wandering attention over and over again is the very root of will. It takes a good deal of effort and discipline. But as one progresses in the practice, less and less effort is needed. The type of attention developed here is anomalous, from the perspective of everyday views of attention: as the stability and vividness of attention increase, the mind becomes more and more relaxed.

According to the Buddhist theory that the stream of consciousness consists of successive moments of cognition, the degree of attentional stability increases in relation to the proportion of ascertaining moments of cognition of the intended object. That is, as stability increases, fewer and fewer moments of ascertaining consciousness are focused on any other object. This makes for a kind of homogeneity of moments of ascertaining perception. The briefest moment of cognition, according to Buddhist psychology, is said to last one to two milliseconds (one sixty-fifth of a finger snap). But in the untrained mind, only a small fraction of these moments of awareness ascertain their object such that one can report on the object afterward. Normally it takes a cluster of successive moments of cognition to achieve recognition of an object. As the vividness, resolution, and brilliance of attention are enhanced, I surmise there must be a greater frequency of moments of ascertaining cognition: the clusters of successive moments that apprehend their object consist of fewer and fewer pulses of cognition. This provides a higher resolution of awareness both over time and in any given moment. In short, Buddhist training of attention results in an exceptionally high density of homogenous moments of ascertaining consciousness.

The Buddhist theoretical understanding of attention and ways to enhance attention skills has considerable relevance for the scientific study of the mind. Before Galileo's construction of the first telescope, many things could not be known about the stars, planets, sun, and moon. Instruments like the telescope were needed for making careful observations of celestial phenomena, and the invention and use of such instruments facilitated the development of the science of astronomy. Without a telescope firmly mounted on a stable platform and finely polished lenses brought into sharp focus, we cannot see whether Jupiter has moons, the sun has spots, the moon has craters, and so forth. We need to look at the phenomena themselves in a stable, precise, clear fashion.

Just as this is true for celestial objects and all other phenomena that are studied scientifically, it is also true for mental phenomena. To develop a comprehensive science of the mind, we must rigorously examine mental phenomena themselves, not just their behavioral and neural correlates. And such a first-person, introspective investigation of the mind must not remain at the level of folk psychology. Individuals engaged in such inquiry must be more highly trained than college undergraduates paid ten dollars an hour to "look at their minds" and report on what they see. Rigorous behavioral and neuroscientific studies of mental processes rely on first-person reports, so to further the progress of the cognitive sciences as a whole, it is important that such observation and reporting not be left to amateurs. The level of sophistication of the first-person study of the mind must rise to the degree of sophistication of the third-person methodologies developed in the behavioral and neurosciences. The science of mind requires the development of something analogous to a telescope, and this need can be filled by the cultivation of refined attention, which allows for stable and vivid observations of mental phenomenon, as Tsongkhapa pointed out 500 years ago.

The scientific study of the mind, in turn, is relevant for Buddhism. Buddhists developed a wide range of techniques for balancing the mind and healing it of afflictive tendencies, including methods for enhancing attention skills. But these techniques were originally created for people living in rural India more than two millennia ago, and then they were adapted for Tibetans over the past 1,200 years. Which Buddhist methods for enhancing attention are most suitable for people living in the modern industrialized world, and to what extent must they be adapted so that they are optimally effective? These are questions with broad relevance not only to Buddhists but to everyone interested in improving attention, and scientific research can be very helpful in finding the answers.

Once attention skills have been enhanced, to what extent can they be transferred to tasks that were not part of the initial training? How durable are these skills? If you rigorously applied yourself to such training—for example, by practicing ten hours each day for months on end—would the enhanced stability and vividness of your attention be retained after you returned to a more normal lifestyle? What are the behavioral and neural correlates of these changes in attention? There is much potential for collaboration here between Buddhist and scientific researchers, with great relevance for improving mental health and education, optimizing human performance, and preventing and treating attention disorders. Buddhism does not have all the answers, but it does provide a wealth of theoretical and practical knowledge that may be of great value to science and society as a whole.

In summary, there is a complementarity between Buddhist and scientific ways of investigating the mind. The forte of Buddhism is its array of first-person methods for directly studying the mind by means of trained, introspective attention. The forte of science is its array of third-person methods for indirectly studying the mind, through rigorous investigation of the neural and behavioral correlates of mental phenomena. The integration of these two approaches is a match waiting to be made, in heaven or at MIT. (Maybe there is not much difference!)

Attention and Cognitive Control

After Jonathan Cohen and Alan Wallace completed their presentations, Arthur Zajonc facilitated a general conversation on the issues and questions they had raised. The speakers and the Dalai Lama were joined by a panel of experts chosen for their different areas of expertise related to the topic in question: Anne Treisman, professor of psychology at Princeton University; David Meyer, professor of psychology at the University of Michigan; and Nancy Kanwisher, professor of brain and cognitive science at MIT and investigator at the McGovern Institute for Brain Research.

ARTHUR ZAJONC: We would now like to return to some of the questions that have been raised. Jonathan asked whether attention can be trained, and about the differences between selective and sustained attention, and between focused and broad attention. Alan looked for occasions for collaboration. We would like to begin by giving the opportunity first to His Holiness to direct his own response to any of these questions, and then we'll turn to our scientific as well as Buddhist colleagues. Your Holiness, do you have something you would like to add at this point?

DALAI LAMA: Jonathan, when you were defining attention in relation to cognitive control and demonstrating some experiments on how quickly one can pay attention to specific features within visual stimuli, it reminded me of certain discussions in classical Buddhist texts about how perception arises and whether there is a multiplicity of perceptions to a stimulus. There is a lot of discussion of this in the Buddhist texts, and in fact there are three different standpoints on this that have some parallel to your discussion of attention. One standpoint asserts that when you are visually confronted with an object, the visual experience itself, coming face to face with the stimuli, is very rich insofar as the sensory faculty is concerned. However, when you pay attention to the object, you can do so selectively. There has been a lot discussion in the Buddhist epistemology as to when perceptions arise. For example, the visual stimuli may include a range of different color combinations. Do the perceptions of these different colors occur simultaneously? Or is perception more like a mirror of what is out there? This second perspective is termed "splitting the egg into half," where the stimuli and the perception are understood to be like two halves of an egg mirroring each other. A third standpoint maintains that, regardless of the diversity and the richness of the stimuli, only one instance of perception occurs when the object comes to attention. This third position seems to be closer to what is suggested by some of the experiments that indicate great selectivity in our attention.

A lot of the experiments that you discussed suggest a level of attention that, from the Buddhist point of view, would be occurring in the domain of thought. The moment you involve cognitive control or some form of selection, you're already at the level of thought rather than sensory experience. In Buddhism, we understand this phenomenon in a very complex way. The initial instance of visual experience occurs at the level of pure sensory experience. There is no evaluative judgment involved, or any discrimination of characteristics. When selection occurs, the attention comes into the picture only at the secondary level of thought. That attention is not really part of the visual experience, from the Buddhist point of view. In fact, from the Buddhist point of view, the object of that attention is not really the visual stimuli. It occurs after the actual experience of the stimuli.

However, attention is considered in Buddhist psychology to be one of the five omnipresent mental factors, which suggests that it is present in all mental experiences. There is a faculty of attention within the field of visual experience itself, so there must be an attention that directs the visual sensory experience to the particular stimuli. You have different levels and categories of attention. It's very complicated. I myself am not very clear on this! *(laughter)*

I spoke of a second level of attention, the level of thought. Another question is whether this attention gives rise to the ascertainment that follows the apprehension of the object. In Buddhist epistemology this is not very clear. We have another set of mental factors known as the five factors of ascertainment, where a level of stability or concentration is required. It is generally understood that this faculty of constant single-pointedness is what gives rise to ascertainment. It's not just attention.

When we speak of these five mental factors of ascertainment, which include aspiration, confidence or trust, mindfulness, single-pointedness, and intelligence, we are not talking about a heightened and trained level of mind. They are naturally occurring faculties that we all experience for a brief period. For example, if there were little or no single-pointed stability in our normal cognitive experience, then we would never be able to apply intelligence. One of the five omnipresent mental factors is known as *sempa*, which could be translated as "will." This is different from aspiration in our system. We are talking here about two different classes of mental factors: five omnipresent factors and five factors of ascertainment. Aspiration is an omnipresent factor; will (sempa) is the other type. But how do you define will, or sempa, as opposed to attention? That is another problem.

ARTHUR ZAJONC: Thank you, Your Holiness. I wonder, Anne, whether you might be able to speak to the question just raised by His Holiness concerning the relation of thought or judgment to attention.

ANNE TREISMAN: In cognitive psychology we've certainly been interested in distinguishing different levels of processing. At the lowest level we have the sensory characteristics of the stimulus. Then, as you move up through different levels, you eventually reach the meaning. But there is some suggestion that, in fact, conscious experience goes directly to the meaning—that we access the highest, conscious level faster than the low levels, and it takes more effort to perceive the sensory properties unchanged by all the interpretations that we spontaneously make.

Another point that is coming to the fore in psychology now and might be relevant is the differentiation between processes that are explicit—that is, information that we are consciously aware of— and processes that are still implicit. We're finding that there may be a great deal of information registered unconsciously in the head. We can show this through evidence of priming, for example. Or, in patients with brain damage who are no longer able to attend to something or to interpret it, we can show that the information has nevertheless gotten into their head somewhere. Attention may involve making explicit information that has already been registered at the sensory level and limiting what we can access consciously.

I wanted to ask the Buddhist philosophers a question: Do you think that you can also expand what you can access consciously at these different levels down to the sensory level, and get away from spontaneous coding at the most cognitive level of meaning, interpretation, and relevance to us?

AJAHN AMARO: Certainly, in the Buddhist tradition, the quality of attention is very definitely seen as something that is trainable and can be developed in very refined ways, as Alan eloquently pointed out. With consistent practice and effort, the mind can usually be trained through focusing on a particularly simple or unified object repeatedly, over many hours, days, weeks, or years, for extended periods of time each day. Capacities to focus at a more and more refined level can then be established quite clearly. Accomplished meditators are known to be able to sustain their attention exclusively on a single object for hours, if not days on end.

ANNE TREISMAN: At what level? In fine sensory detail or active associations or. . . ?

AJAHN AMARO: It would depend on the object, and also on the decision of the person who is focusing. You can choose to have an extremely refined or somewhat broader focus. In attending to things at a refined level, some people are certainly capable of ascertaining the difference between the sense contact, for instance of a color, and where the mind perceives, even before naming it, that this is green or this is red. Obviously not everyone is able to do that, but the more deeply developed the meditation is, the quicker you are in the process. The mapping of the perceptual process is understood in terms of the eye and light coming together. The two form what in Buddhist psychology is called eye consciousness. Those three together (eye, light, and eye consciousness) then condition feeling through an initial percept of attractive, unattractive, or neutral feeling. Then the *saññā,* or designation, occurs. Prior to naming, the brain says, "Oh, this is a color, and it's of this particular intensity." The naming or thought element comes in subsequent to that. Given refined training, the attention can be sustained at that contact level.

ARTHUR ZAJONC: David, did you want to add something?

DAVID MEYER: I wanted to mention that, in this day and age, we have a quite different kind of problem as well. We don't need to sustain our attention so much as we need to shift it back and forth very often. In current times, people are suffering from a disorder I call MAD, and by that I do not mean angry. I mean they are suffering from multitasking addiction disorder. *(laughter)*

ARTHUR ZAJONC: That's a piece of jargon we need to translate for His Holiness. *(laughter)*

DAVID MEYER: I'm sure Your Holiness is quite familiar with this in your own life. Even this weekend, you will need to change back and forth between a variety of activities, one after the other, very quickly. Possibly this is driving you "MAD": you are developing multitasking addiction disorder. You have to do too many tasks all at the same time. The question, both from the scientific perspective and from the spiritual or contemplative perspective, is how to deal with this in modern life. We are inundated with cell phones, the Internet, computers, and I don't know what other gadgets you have right there—there are at least three or four of them. They are all causing us great headaches. *(laughter)*

We scientists have tried to approach this topic by understanding in more detail what takes place in the mind and the brain while people are trying to cope with multitasking. Our research is primarily experimental in nature, but it leads to the theoretical standpoint that there are executive mental processes in the mind, somewhat like a chief executive officer of a big company. These processes are responsible for allocating the mind's resources—memory, attention, perception, and so forth—to deal with one task or another, either at the same time or in rapid succession, much like we are doing right here. The audience out there is trying to listen to us, watch the screen, talk to their friends, and do many other things.

How do we know these executive processes that allocate our mental resources are present, and what is their nature? We have been conducting experiments in which we ask people to perform two or more tasks at the same time, somewhat like talking on a cell phone and driving, or like trying to write a report while being constantly interrupted by telephone calls. We have been measuring people's behavior, including how quickly and how accurately they are able to perform the tasks at the same time. We find that under many conditions, depending on what the tasks are, individuals have great difficulty in doing this so-called multitasking, at least at first. For example, we take an individual such as Jonathan here and give him a couple of very easy tasks to do. Jonathan, when I hold up my fingers, tell me how many there are. Can you do that?

David holds up four fingers.

JONATHAN COHEN: Four.
DAVID MEYER. That's excellent. What about this?

He holds up two fingers.

JONATHAN COHEN: Two.
DAVID MEYER: Good. This is a visual task involving a verbal response. Now let's give you another task. If I go "beep," I want you to say "high." And if I go "boop," I want you to say "low." Can you do that?
JONATHAN COHEN: I can try.

David pronounces a string of "beeps" and "boops" to much laughter from the audience, and Jonathan responds appropriately with "high" or "low."

DAVID MEYER: Now I want you to do it really fast.

David speeds up the exercise, and Jonathan's responses keep up with him. The audience reacts with laughter and applause.

JONATHAN COHEN: There are other subjects available, you know! Our Buddhist friends were afraid that we were going to ask them to be the guinea pigs. *(laughter)*
DAVID MEYER: He's actually doing pretty well, folks, but he's had

prior training. This is one of our major discoveries. It's very difficult at first, especially when the tasks conflict with each other, for example because they both involve language. Even using a cell phone while driving is difficult, despite what the automobile and telephone companies would like you to believe. Driving involves talking to yourself. You have to read signs. You have to think about what you want to do next when you're in traffic, and so on. We find that performance in terms of speed and accuracy is very poor under those circumstances. But with appropriate practice and training, we can get people to develop strategies for multitasking that make their executive mental processes more efficient. It is possible, as a result of such training, to overcome differences that exist between people in their ability to multitask.

This raises a number of interesting questions from the scientific perspective that could feed directly into insights and wisdom provided by contemplative traditions like Buddhism. What would the Buddhist perspective tell not only the scientists but also the public about how they should deal with this MAD, multitasking addiction disorder? Or OCD—online compulsive disorder? *(laughter)* What is to be done, not only from the scientific perspective but also from the Buddhist perspective, if what's wanted now is not necessarily sustained focus of the attention on one object, but rather the ability to switch effortlessly back and forth between one task and another?

ALAN WALLACE: The training of focusing on a single object is preparation for using the attention in a myriad of other ways. In fact, multitasking occurs in a wide variety of other Buddhist meditative techniques, many of them in Tibetan Buddhism. You may be performing some ritual action with your hands, chanting verbally, and engaging in a complex, multifaceted visualization, all at the same time. You might be multitasking across these different channels over a period of an hour, or as long as ten hours. That is a common practice.

JONATHAN COHEN: Alan, are there specific practices that focus on that particular ability, or is that something you encounter but with no particular training dedicated to it?

ALAN WALLACE: You develop those abilities by engaging in this type of multitasking meditative practice. You may, if you wish, engage in a more simple meditative practice first, focusing on a single, simple object, honing stability and vividness. Then at some point you might shift over to much more complex meditative practices. But some people choose not to do the preliminary practice. They will develop the stability and vividness in the course of the more complex practice.

JONATHAN COHEN: Can I infer that the same applies here as in learning more focused abilities—that initially it's hard, but ultimately you come to a state where you can multitask with greater relaxation and comfort? That would seem to imply some therapeutic interventions for MAD and OCD. *(laughter)*

AJAHN AMARO: Generally these two qualities are developed in parallel and they support each other. In Buddhist jargon, one is called concentration practice, specifically focusing on a single object. The other we might call mindfulness, which usually develops more of an all-around sense of the moment and what's going on. It applies not only to a particular religious practice, as Alan was talking about, but also to the normal flow of life in a monastery. Often when you meet a great master like His Holiness, or other great teachers that I have known, you are astonished by how they can be in a group of people and be serving eight or ten different people in different ways simultaneously. They are actually attending to the needs and particular responses from several people all at the same time, and each individual will have a sense of being perfectly attended to.

It is most interesting that, from the subjective point of view of the person who is speaking, they are not thinking, "I'm going to take care of that one. And what about this one? And, oh dear, that one over there." Rather, the more that mindfulness and concentration are developed, the more this practice flows naturally. It is not forced, so it's not exhausting to multitask. It's not even really burdensome, for someone who is very accomplished and experienced.

DAVID MEYER: Would you say that after developing this ability you can actually do various tasks simultaneously without conflict between them, as if you were doing only one?

AJAHN AMARO: I would think so. It depends tremendously on the attitude with which you approach it. You phrased it "the multitasking addictive disorder," but I would say that the addiction is different from the multitasking. *(applause)*

NANCY KANWISHER: I am very happy to hear that I can stay on e-mail all the time!

I wanted to go back to the temporal structure of awareness that Alan mentioned briefly. It is also relevant to this issue of multitasking. There is quite a lot of work being done now in cognitive neuroscience on the rate and temporal properties of perceptual and cognitive processing. There is evidence that people can recognize an object in about a tenth of a second, or maybe two-tenths of a second. You can present a rapid sequence of completely unrelated, complex scenes to people at a rate of eight per second, and they will extract the gist of each one more or less accurately. There is also work showing that although people are often aware of each item in a sequence at that presentation rate, under some circumstances some items simply fail to enter awareness at all. There is reason to believe they get processed in some way but fail to enter awareness.

I was fascinated to hear the notion that a moment is ten milliseconds. Is that consistent? Where does that come from, and how does it fit?

ALAN WALLACE: There is a notion in Buddhism that cognition consists of a sequence of pulses of cognition. While I've used the term "one millisecond," of course Tibetans did not have precise watches to measure it. What they did was take the duration of a snap of a finger, divide that by sixty-five, and call this "a moment." I have heard some discussion that a single moment of cognition may be one sixty-fourth of the duration of a fingersnap; it probably depends on the thickness of the thumb. *(laughter)* Be that as it may, if a finger snap is roughly a tenth of a second, and you divide it by sixty-five, that comes to roughly one millisecond.

Having said that, the Buddhist position is that a single millisecond of cognition almost invariably does not ascertain anything by itself. It is too brief. But in a sequence of these pulses of cognition, if they are focusing on the same object with a high degree of homogeneity, a temporal binding process takes place and there is a cumulative effect. And after a multitude of these milliseconds, whether ten or forty or a hundred, then you ascertain the object you are attending to.

I would offer a hypothesis, that for this type of attentional training, as you enhance the clarity of attention, which I understand to mean increasing the density of these ascertaining clusters of consciousness, you would be able to pick up things of shorter duration and also pick up more detail in a single moment. In other words, vividness corresponds in part to the degree of temporal resolution, the ability to ascertain very brief stimuli. That is a hypothesis that is just waiting to be tested.

NANCY KANWISHER: What kinds of things do people report when they ascertain these ten-millisecond moments? Is there anything that can be said about it, or is this necessarily just first-person? If you reach this insight, can you share it with anybody?

AJAHN AMARO: Some of the brain-imaging techniques, the work of Richard Davidson and others, that I have been shown in the past couple of days have got me thinking that maybe you can measure this from the outside, but it is generally subjective experience. It is said that the Buddha's most senior disciple, Sariputta, was supposed to be such an accomplished meditator, so skilled at concentration and attentive abilities, that he could track not only each individual mind moment but the seventeen different parts of an individual mind moment. When the Buddha asked him to describe how he experienced this in very deep concentration, he laid out the pattern of events as he experienced them. The Buddha said, "It is as if you've taken a cup full of water and described where each of the molecules of the water came from. It is well done, Sariputta." I don't know whether you can actually measure that from the outside with one of these wonderful gadgets here at MIT or in Wisconsin. But certainly individuals report this and can describe their experience.

DALAI LAMA: In Buddhist psychology there is a recognition of what one could call laws of psychology. Compared with characteristics and properties of the body, mental states are thought to have certain unique characteristics, one of which is that, through constant familiarity and habituation, mental states can be enhanced and developed further. So that is one important feature. Another important feature is that mental states and characteristics are thought to be more stable than physical characteristics. It is on the basis of these two premises, in Buddhist psychology and epistemology, that there is an understanding that many of the mental states can be trained and enhanced.

It was time now, Arthur Zajonc decided, to open the floor to questions from the audience. Earlier, audience members had been instructed to write any questions they had on slips of paper and leave them in the aisles to be collected and carried up to the stage. This had been done, and Anne Harrington—who was off duty as moderator in this session and would serve as the voice of the audience by reading the questions—had begun to sift through the first batch.

ARTHUR ZAJONC: Let's turn to one of the audience questions.
ANNE HARRINGTON: I have three: one is for the Buddhists and one for the scientists, and one is for both. I'm going to start with the last. Here is what the questioner asks: "A teenager can be totally attentive on a second-by-second level and yet be both relaxed and enjoying the experience for hours. We call this video gaming. *(laughter)* The same teenager has difficulty with attention at school. So does it follow that the real question for attention researchers, the key question," says this member of the audience, "is

how to enhance the study of attention to boring stimuli?" *(laughter and applause)*

NANCY KANWISHER: There's a recent study by a cognitive psychologist named Daphne Bavelier, who has shown that, in fact, video game playing can lead to surprisingly powerful benefits in visual attention in very different tasks. This is something that many of us in the field did not expect. I don't know if it's what the questioner wanted to hear, but the effects are quite striking.

DAVID MEYER: I'm not sure that I buy into the idea that tasks whose performance we study in the lab are entirely boring. In many respects we try to create situations in the lab that are much like playing video games. We provide appropriate reinforcement and encouragement for good performance. Often the people we study tell us afterward that they would be willing to pay to come back and do it again. I think we wind up being able to reach conclusions about the nature of attention and control not only in the performance of boring tasks, but also in the performance of ones that are similar to what you have in real life with activities like video game playing.

ALAN WALLACE: In the disciplined training of the attention, you tend to focus on a single object or a process, such as breathing. For the first fifteen seconds or so, it might be quite interesting. Then after that you may say, "If you've seen one breath, you've seen them all." I personally find video games very boring. How interesting something is depends not simply on the quality of the object but on our relationship to it. I have spent a fair amount of time attending to the breath, and not just because I have a penchant for breathing but because there is a higher order of interest in it. After a while, even if the respiration (or some generated mental image that you are focusing on as your reference for stabilizing the attention) is not interesting objectively, there is a higher-order level of interest based on anticipated benefits. It's rather like slogging through medical school for four years. It can't all be interesting all the time, but you are anticipating the benefits you and others will get out of it, and this holds your attention.

DAVID MEYER: Exactly. In fact we find that, by providing appropriate feedback in the lab, people get very involved in monitoring the progress of their own performance and the acquisition of higher-order levels of skill. This provides a self-sustaining motive to continue doing it, even though some of these tasks, at a lower level, might be construed as being quite boring.

ALAN WALLACE: That monitoring process itself can be fascinating.

ARTHUR ZAJONC: This comes back to the meta-attention that you brought up.

AJAHN AMARO: I think there is a mixture of things happening. Certainly, attention skills might be developed through repetitious activity and fine-tuning of focus in a task such as playing video games, which may be why they increase skills in certain academic areas. But the element of habituation has another side. The way films are made, the average clip is very, very brief, just a few seconds long. What that means is one gets bored more easily. If you need a high level of rapidly changing stimuli to keep your attention, then as soon as things drop below that level, you are bored. You want to do something new, something different. So there are two contrasting elements involved in that habituation. Teenagers, or even adults, might be harmed by repetitious, high-intensity activity if it leads to a need for so much stimulus coming in just to avoid feeling depressed or restless.

One purpose of learning to develop attention with uninteresting objects like the breath is to establish that quality of attention and ease with the present moment with an absolute minimum of stimuli, so that you can feel at home in yourself with very little going on. Teenagers need to be playing a video game and listening to the stereo and checking their e-mail simultaneously, and then they feel good! That takes a lot of hardware to feel at home in life.

ARTHUR ZAJONC: Perhaps you can tell that Ajahn is a forest monk.

AJAHN AMARO: I also have an iPod. *(laughter)*

ANNE HARRINGTON: Here is another question from the audience, and it is primarily directed to His Holiness. Alan gave a lucid summary of Gelugpa mind training vis-à-vis attention, but other methods of mental cultivation and other schools of Tibetan Buddhism may be equally relevant to the cultivation of attention. Are mantra practices relevant, or ritual practices in which deities are visualized and interacted with? How might these understandings be incorporated into this conversation about attentional training?

DALAI LAMA: The perspective that we are bringing to the discussion here is from the common tradition of Buddhist psychology known as Abhidharma. Within that, the Tibetan tradition recognizes two different systems of Abhidharma, the upper and lower. In regard to mantra recitation, the very meditation manual that gives the mantra recitation contains an explicit statement that a practitioner who is wearied after meditation should then engage in the recitation of mantras. So in a strict sense, the mantra recitation is not part of the actual meditation. Of course, in the process of training the attention, attention can be applied to different focuses. It could be applied to some external material object or to mental processes, or to the nature of the mind itself, or it could be used to visualize certain imagery.

ANNE HARRINGTON: Continuing with questions from the audience, I have one that seems to be intended for Jonathan Cohen. It reads: "Buddhist meditation involves training attentional capacities. Psychology assumes that subjects have no particular attentional training. If you had access to a pool of subjects highly trained in attention, how might you use them in your research paradigm? What new questions could you ask or begin to answer?"

JONATHAN COHEN: There are all kinds of phenomenally interesting claims that have been made about Buddhist practice that are relevant here. How quickly can one switch one's attention? We have made measurements under certain circumstances but with naive subjects. How much can one exceed the capacity to switch that we have measured so far, when appropriate training has been given to the subject? The claim that Ajahn made earlier, that one could direct attention to the very earliest stages of processing, perhaps earlier than we have been able to measure in naive subjects, is interesting to us. How early in the stream?

I'll be quite honest: there was a great temptation when I came to this meeting to view the Buddhists as guinea pigs. I sense that at least a couple of my colleagues initially had this same attitude. We had heard all these incredible claims and we were tempted at first to say, "Let's get them in the laboratory and start measuring these things." But the Buddhists wanted to talk about theory and philosophy as well. It was almost as if we were interested in psychophysics and were going to study major-league pitchers: we wanted to understand how they threw the ball fast, and they wanted to explain the philosophy behind it, which had to do with which way they point their shoes in the locker before the game. We wanted to say, "Look, I'll figure out how it happens. You just do it for me."

For myself, and I think this is true for all of us, the most gratifying part of this experience is disabusing ourselves of that narrowness of mind and realizing that there are some very interesting ideas that stand behind the claims. And so I would like to turn the question on its head and say, "I can think of a million things to measure, but I'm interested in what *you* think would be the right things to measure." *(applause)* That would instruct us as much in our perspective as it would allow us to understand yours better. We would like to hear what the Buddhists are interested in measuring and why. What would you gain by making these measurements?

ALAN WALLACE: I would like to see something very practical come out of the research, especially in terms of mental health. In the West there is a marvelous science of mental illness, but once you get to normal, you are pretty much shunted out the door. You have reached the level of a psychiatrist, and if you improved any more it might be embarrassing for your therapist. It would be good to have a clear vision of what mental health is—exceptional mental health at the upper end of the spectrum—and practical strategies for developing mental balance way beyond normal. We know what it is like to be physically normal, but we also have Olympic athletes. What would it be like to have an Olympic status of mental health? What would be the constituent parts? I would love to see that studied.

AJAHN AMARO: In Buddhist philosophy, one is not considered sane until one is fully enlightened; so the bar is set in a slightly different place.

JONATHAN COHEN: But how will the tools of modern science help us better understand how to get there? What specific experiments could we do that would inform Buddhist practice and help improve that?

AJAHN AMARO: In looking at brain-scan images yesterday, one of the interesting possibilities that came to mind was to study the effects of one's behavior, and particularly the ethical quality of one's lifestyle and its relation to positive self-image. One's sense of comfort in life and connection with others is associated with the way that one lives and how honest one is or how prone to acting violently or aggressively. In all of these different studies, I haven't seen that kind of ethical element. I know there is a great urge to separate the ethical element from research, but as His Holiness often points out, ethics is not confined to religion. It is a natural human quality and it has a powerful effect. I would like to see research that could demonstrate very clearly, medically and psychologically, that living an ethical lifestyle—not acting harmfully, being honest, and so forth—genuinely improves the quality of life, no matter what age you are, from early childhood on up.

NANCY KANWISHER: It sounds to me like you are advocating a study of the neural correlates of wholesome behavior or an ethical lifestyle. As a neuroscientist, that seems of some interest, but I am curious about what you would get out of that. After all, you don't need our pretty brain pictures to decide what kind of life you want to live.

AJAHN AMARO: What I get out of it is a healthier world and the delight of humanity being in a better state than it was before.

NANCY KANWISHER: How does neuroscience, specifically, contribute to that?

AJAHN AMARO: Because people believe in the great god of data.

NANCY KANWISHER: So it is a public relations tool?

ARTHUR ZAJONC: You might say it is the validation of a tenet within Buddhism that is perhaps viewed with a certain amount of uncertainty, at least, by others. Perhaps that is not a sufficient motivation for scientists to get involved?

ALAN WALLACE: As William James recognized, first-person reports are prone to error, like any other report. We make errors about our own subjective experiences, and yet we are extremely confident about them. In a contemplative setting you have some checks and balances. You go to your teacher and report, and sometimes your teacher says: "What you said in that self-report is wrong. I'm observing you from a second-person perspective as a mentor, and I have to correct you." So there is a dialogue. But sometimes the mentor may be wrong. Assuming that the mentor is not clairvoyant, if we have some psychological and neuroscientific measures, it is as if, metaphorically, we develop a three-dimensional perspective, vectoring from three different perspectives to give us greater confidence in what's going on. That could be enormously helpful for contemplatives, and generally in spiritual practice, to evaluate how we are doing.

DAVID MEYER: It seems there is a real possibility of a feedback loop between first-person and third-person perspectives in which, for example, the first-person perspective could provide direct evidence that a third-person measurement is a manifestation of a particular desirable or undesirable mental state. We could then investigate, through certain kinds of training and practice, what it takes to move closer to that apparent state. In the course of that investigation, especially once that state has been reached by someone who was not there before, it may be possible for that person to report back and verify, from the first-person perspective, that they have in fact moved from one place to another. And around and around you go. For this to take place, individuals coming from different approaches would have to be engaged in the overall synthesis.

ARTHUR ZAJONC: That's right. There is an opportunity and a value in the collaboration.

DALAI LAMA: Jonathan's presentation and the subsequent discussion reminded me of the ancient debate among Buddhist epistemologists over three models: the egg split in half, one instance of percept with a multiplicity of objects, and percepts equal in number and parallel to the richness of the stimuli. There has been a lot of debate on these three perspectives, but there doesn't seem to have been any real settlement. My curiosity has been raised by the possibility of using modern scientific instruments and methods to determine who is right. *(laughter)*

ARTHUR ZAJONC: All of our curiosities have been stimulated, and I think we have already begun to develop the spirit of collaboration we have been hoping for.

III

IMAGERY
AND
VISUALIZATION

Buddhist Perspectives on Mental Imagery

I wish to explain a few things about how mental imagery is used in Buddhist practice as a tool serving the effort to achieve personal transformation. You may wonder why Buddhists spend so much time trying to visualize images. We need to place these efforts in a larger perspective. They are part of a more general goal of achieving a transformation of the way we perceive the phenomenal world as well as the way we conceive of the nature of the perceiver—the "I," the subject.

Why do we need to transform these things? What is wrong with the way in which we ordinarily perceive the world? Usually when we perceive the world, we cannot help but assign to it values and judgments. In some cases, of course, doing so helps us to function in this world. If we know something is very hot, we need to be careful with it. If we know that something is dangerous, we keep our distance. But the process quickly solidifies, and soon we start assigning or imputing characteristics to external objects that we feel are intrinsic to them but are not. We might think this floor is beautiful because we perceive it as such. But very quickly we tend to believe that it is intrinsically beautiful, or ugly. We believe that sounds are intrinsically pleasant or unpleasant, and so, similarly, in the cases of taste, touch, and all our sensory experiences. In fact, there is a deeply interdependent process between outer phenomena and our mind. We perceive things and assign values to them; we try to possess things or discard them based on those judgments; and we start to believe that the characteristics we impute to objects actually belong to the objects. In this way, we experience a much stronger compulsion to attract or repulse them.

The problem is that our experiences of craving or repulsion are at odds with reality. Things are not intrinsically beautiful or pleasant. A rose might be beautiful to our eyes, but its "beauty" does not mean much to a whale or a bat. Because our perception is at odds with reality, we end up with a sense of frustration, torment, inner conflict, and suffering. Likewise for the perceiver's experience of him- or herself. We know that our body changes from that of a baby to that of an adult to that of an elderly person. We know, too, that in our experience every moment brings something new. Yet we can't help but think that in this stream of constant transformation there is a core, the I, which defines us, which is *really* us, and which continues in a unitary way throughout this process. This is our instinctive belief. Once we have this core identification with an I, obviously we want to protect it and please it. Feelings of fear, rejection, or attraction are connected with the strong sense of self-importance that comes from believing in this I. The same sense of self-importance also provides a target to suffering. Through identification with the core I, we become very vulnerable to all kinds of emotional afflictions: intense craving, hatred, pride, contempt, and jealousy. Jealousy, for instance, could not exist without a sense of self-importance as its cause.

In Buddhist thinking, such experiences are considered *deluded perceptions*, because in such perceptions we are solidifying both the inner reality of the stream of consciousness (which is constantly changing) and the flow of ever-changing phenomena outside. Imputing or superimposing our judgments, likes, and dislikes onto phenomena to an excessive extent causes us to place tremendous importance on the self and in this way actually makes us function in a way that causes torment and suffering. The whole idea of the Buddhist path is to acknowledge and recognize that suffering and its causes for what they are. This is the answer to the question of what's wrong with our way of perceiving the phenomenal world: it's just wrong in the sense that it ends up in suffering and torment. That torment in turn prevents us from being open to others and expressing altruism.

If we could remedy our tendency toward deluded perceptions, it would definitely be a step toward understanding the true nature of reality: this in turn would help us to stop clinging to it as something solid, but instead to recognize the illusory nature of our conception of the perceiver as a unitary, distinct entity within. This recognition does not result in a loss of identity. Instead, one wins inner freedom in relation to phenomena and to the stream of one's thoughts.

This is the larger context for the use within Buddhist practice of mental imagery. Imagery offers a skillful means of replacing "impure," deluded perceptions—which attach strong characteristics to the objects of the phenomenal world—with a much more "fluid" attitude that is attuned to the ever-changing stream of consciousness.

The use of mental imagery in Buddhist practice is also grounded in a particular understanding of the nature of mind and its relation to destructive or obscuring emotions. From the Buddhist perspective, it is believed that when you look deep within the mind, you come to a perception of pure consciousness. This is the continuum that Buddhists sometimes call the "luminous aspect of mind": a pure cognitive faculty that is free of any mental constructs or images. We believe that this basic luminosity does not intrinsically contain anger, jealousy, pride, contempt, or disgust. Instead, all those mental factors evolve out of our grasping, which is in turn caused by our deluded way of perceiving reality. The process of gaining freedom from frustration and torment requires that we become more introspectively aware of the basic nature of consciousness, so that we can free ourselves from the obscuring emotions that arise out of this cognitive faculty.

Those understandings inform the way mental imagery, or visualization, is used in Buddhist meditative practice. When we are attached in different ways to the phenomenal world, and attached also to ourselves and our ways of relating to others, we end up with a certain perception of our body, our name, our mind, the various things that we believe characterize ourselves, the I. Most of us have been functioning within the framework of these perceptions for a long time. Generating mental images is one way to remind ourselves of— or bring ourselves closer to—what Buddhists believe to be the true nature of mind. Under normal circumstances, most of us are constantly following a deluded chain of thoughts, each associated with a charge of attraction or repulsion that in turn gives rise to further such experiences, until the mind is completely invaded and enslaved by disturbing thoughts. If, however, we can harness this constant movement of the mind and turn its attention to something that will slowly bring us back to our true nature, we may be able to break out of that process.

To achieve this purpose, we use images with symbolic meaning. For instance, we know that we have two arms that we use for different activities. We can play badminton with them, which is a fine thing to do, but it's also a limited use of our arms. So to extend our sense of possibilities, we visualize ourselves as a particular deity, using representations that may seem strange—four or more arms, or three heads. In so doing, the point is to remember and focus on the meaning of the image. Two arms in Buddhist thinking represent the pairing of wisdom (the understanding of reality) and compassion (the expression of wisdom). Four arms symbolize boundless love, boundless compassion, boundless rejoicing, and boundless equanimity. If we visualize a form possessed of six arms, this symbolizes the perfection of discipline, generosity, diligence, concentration, wisdom, and patience. Likewise, a form with three heads symbolizes the transformation of the three main mental toxins: hatred, craving, and mental delusion or lack of discernment. Having visualized these attributes for ourselves, we then go on to visualize them for other beings in the same way, and for our environment more generally.

In a way, doing this kind of task may seem somewhat artificial and to be taking us even further away from reality. But in fact we are trying to transform our perception of the world from a delusional perception into one that constantly reminds us of the basic quality of pure awareness when it is free from obscuring emotions. Most of us have a strongly engrained habit of perceiving solid characteristics in objects. We are like pieces of paper that have been rolled up for a long time; if you spread them flat on a table and take your hands away, they will roll up again. It takes time to replace engrained mental tendencies with more free perceptions that take into account interdependence, the ultimate nature of reality, and the true nature of mind.

So this is why we use mental imagery, to help us achieve such perceptions. The process involves systematic training. An individual might, for instance, take as the object of his concentration an image of a Buddha, or a deity with symbolic attributes. Initially he will train the attention by looking very carefully at the details of an actual, external representation of the image. He will then try to recreate the image internally in the absence of the representation. He will cultivate his abilities over a long period. For instance, during several weeks of day-long training, he might spend a session of three hours concentrating on the black and white shape of the eyes, according to the harmonious proportions that we see in representations of the Buddha. Then he will move to other details, the specific oval shape of the face, the specific way of sitting, et cetera, and spend a great deal of time on each of these. If he's working with a more complex representation than the Buddha Shakyamuni—a deity with multiple arms and heads and specific ornaments, for instance—he might spend a whole session on a particular set of ornaments or clothing, going over each detail one by one, from the top to the bottom and again from the bottom to the top, spending time on each detail.

He will also practice the skill of bringing the mind back when it wanders. In a fashion similar to what happens when one concentrates on any object of attention, attention may slip away from what one is trying to visualize in two ways. The mind may become distracted, in which case one tries to become aware of the fact that one's mind has wandered and bring the attention back gently to where it belongs, like a butterfly leaving a flower and then coming back to it. Alternatively, the mind may sink into torpor, lassitude, and fatigue, and the visualization may consequently become dim and unclear. In such a case, there are ways to bring back or revive the attention, or, alternatively, one can take a rest before coming back to the task refreshed. The point is that one repeats processes like these over and over. When we have become familiar with each and every detail of the representation, we can start to form a more global image of what we're trying to visualize. After a while, the image as a whole becomes clearer.

It is said that there are three goals to visualization, each of which needs to be achieved step by step. The first is *clarity*: the faculty to see clearly the minutest detail of the image. There are different methods we can use to increase our capacity for clarity. For example, instead of visualizing a deity the same size as our own body, we might instead visualize it as big as a mountain, and then walk around the details of the visualization as if we were a deer moving through and across that mountain. Alternatively we may do just the opposite: make the deity as small as a sesame seed but try to keep the visualization very clear and still mentally retain all the details. We thus exercise our visualization in many different ways, changing the deity, moving it around, looking at it from different perspectives, until we have a consistently clear perception.

The second goal of training is to become precisely aware at all times of the *meaning* of what we are visualizing, because visualization as an end in itself doesn't lead us anywhere. If we remind ourselves, for instance, that the deity's two arms represent the qualities of wisdom and compassion, then slowly the usual stream of deluded thoughts and self-centeredness will be replaced by these qualities. This conclusion is based on a very simple observation: you cannot at the same time shake someone's hand in a friendly manner and give him a blow. You can do both in two separate gestures, but not both at the same time. Similarly, you cannot feel hatred and love at the same moment toward the same object. You can alternate between the two, but you cannot feel both in the very same moment. It follows, therefore, that the more the mind is occupied with such qualities as altruism, patience, and inner peace, the less space their opposites—hatred, animosity, craving, jealousy, and so forth—have to occupy the mind.

A third goal of training is to rediscover one's true nature and gain *confidence* in the new way of perceiving things that one has cultivated. Through visualization, we come to realize that our cravings, our clinging to external objects we have decided are beautiful or desirable, and repelling those we find ugly or offensive—that all these experiences are fabrications of our mind. The qualities don't truly exist in the object. If we can realize this, we will experience much more inner freedom in our relationship to the phenomenal world. Similarly, if I visualize myself as a deity or as the Buddha Shakyamuni for a few months, it really helps me to improve a little bit and begin to cultivate some of the qualities that are fully developed in the Buddha. Fifty-eight years of visualizing myself as just myself, a French monk with a big nose and big belly, didn't help me much.

We call this goal of visualization "wisdom pride": not in the sense of being proud in an ordinary way of being the Buddha, but simply in the sense of feeling the confidence that comes from rediscovering the true nature of our mind, free from obscuring emotions. That rediscovery is the only way to achieve genuine inner peace and happiness. The confidence one experiences contrasts powerfully with the usual whirlpool of hopes and fears that fill our mind when we invest all our hope in things outside ourselves. We think that if we could arrange the outer world in a certain way we would be happy; or we think that, when things go wrong, we could get rid of our suffering if we could manipulate the outer circumstances. It never works. We need instead to look at the inner conditions of genuine flourishing, which have to do with our state of mind.

When we begin such visualizations, we first imagine dissolving our ordinary body into light and emptiness. We imagine our mind having the same nature as that of the deity we're trying to visualize. In this way, we learn to rediscover our true nature. We are not trying to make reality more complicated or artificial. We are just using a skillful means of rediscovering our true nature.

How do great contemplatives describe the experience of stabilizing the image and making it clearer? They say that at the first stage, it is just a mental construct. The visualization has been, by that time, built up step by step through perhaps four sessions a day, each lasting three hours. This represents a very intense engagement with the process of generating images with all their symbolic meaning. Nevertheless, at this stage it is still definitely a mental construct. To get a more stable image, they must continue to work on the visualization. They're not trying to visualize something solid, because in fact that's what they want to avoid. So they try instead to see the image more as if it were made of light, as if it were a very, very clear rainbow. It is not made of flesh and blood or wood or stone. It is also, however, not inert as a rainbow is. And it has the qualities of wisdom and compassion, so it acts to remind and inspire contemplatives to let those inner qualities flourish within their mind.

The image may continue to feel artificial for a long time, but it is said that when the contemplative gains mastery over the visualization process, it becomes effortless. Indeed, it is said that at a certain point in time the visualization can "arise to the sense organs" like a truly perceived object and without effort. When some meditators think of the image of the Buddha or a deity, the image then just comes, almost like an object seen in reality, although they know that what they are seeing is in their mind. It is described as emerging in all its clarity, all its vividness, all its stability, like a "fish leaping out of water." Complete and clear, natural and effortless, it simply appears.

One might say that what we have here has to do with a type of conditioning, or with a fabricated image that one is powerless to control. An important part of the training at this point, however, is to arrive at a point at which one is able to let the image vanish without leaving any trace, in just the same way as one was able initially to generate it.

Of course there exist some people who have not undergone any meditative training, who also have described experiences of visions that appear very clearly and without apparent effort. I read about someone who thought that his dog came into the operating room when his brain was stimulated in a certain way during surgery. Apparently that person saw the dog just as clearly as I might see something truly in front of me—a pot of flowers, say. It seems, though, that in the case of the hallucinated dog we are dealing with a pathological state. This is very different, I think, from the kinds of visualizations that result from training in people whose minds are extremely healthy, and who, by any other consideration, are very stable, peaceful, and reliable.

In sum, visualization really helps one to achieve a very profound mastery of the workings of the mind. The rationale for training to a point at which you can stabilize mental images is not to encourage one to get caught up in the content of an internal movie filled with three-dimensional Buddha fields and so on. It's to give one access to inner freedom, to a state in which one is no longer attached to a view of the phenomenal world as so solid; a state in which one no longer superimposes the qualities of pleasant, unpleasant, ugly, or disgusting on that world; a state in which one also experiences much more inner freedom in relationship to the perceiver—not believing in the solid permanence of this "I," Matthieu Ricard, who perceived those delusional categories for so many years. Where one arrives instead is at a place where one realizes the interdependence that exists between the stream of consciousness—which is like a continuously flowing river (but without the boat of the ego floating on it)—and ceaselessly changing phenomena. One appreciates the relationship among all phenomena that we normally solidify as being separate entities. All the frustrations and torments that come from solidifying both the external world and the perceiver also disappear. One does not become like a vegetable, indifferent to everything, but at the same time one is no longer caught in all the attractions and repulsions that come precisely from a false perception of reality. Freedom from torments means inner peace, which is quite different from the effort to find happiness in external phenomena and the fleeting pleasures and sensations they produce. That sense of inner peace, in turn, naturally brings much more openness to the world and other sentient beings. Lack of fear, lack of self-importance or self-identity naturally flourish, along with greater altruism, compassion, and loving kindness, because the barriers between self and others have been removed.

Unless one understands the goals of such a practice, it will seem very odd that one might spend six months or more trying to visualize a very complex image. And, indeed, not only do people involved in this practice seek to visualize single deities but some also seek to visualize mandalas, which are assemblies of deities that may be more than 700 in number. Meditators exist who can visualize all 700 deities in detail, one after the other. People like that show the kind of capacity that one can develop.

The process, taken as a whole, is like climbing a ladder. Once you have climbed to the roof with the ladder, you don't need to take the ladder up on your back. Complex visualizations like these are extremely profound meditation techniques for transforming one's self. Eventually they lead to an understanding of the deep nature of one's mind, the pure consciousness that is free from obscuring emotions. When this is understood, one is much more free and better equipped for life; when thoughts and emotions do arise, they don't invade one's mind and enslave one's passions. The freedom that results is one of the secrets of genuine and lasting happiness.

STEPHEN M. KOSSLYN, DANIEL REISBERG,
AND MARLENE BEHRMANN

Introspection and Mechanism in Mental Imagery

We want to focus on the relation between what is evident to introspection, the process of "looking within," and the mechanisms that underlie mental imagery.[1] Introspection is one way to learn about mental imagery, but how accurate is this method, either in telling us about imagery itself or in telling us about the mechanisms that underlie mental imagery? As we will see, this question receives a mixed answer, because introspection is richly informative about some aspects of imagery but less so about others.

We would like to start off by pointing out that we will be assessing introspection by comparing its results to the results of laboratory studies, and, without question, one must be aware of the limitations of such laboratory studies. Buddhist tradition has produced a remarkable body of reports about imagery, with enormous scope, depth, and subtlety. Learning about these observations should remind us how little we in the scientific community know about imagery, just how narrow and focused we've been. The scientific community, here as elsewhere, has made progress by focusing first on a narrow, simplified set of phenomena, with the intention of then examining how the lessons learned in this way can be applied to a broader, more realistic set of real-world observations. We hope that we are starting to make a few bricks that can contribute to the wall, but we really must be modest in any claims we make during this very early stage of our research.

With that preface, we would like to summarize briefly some key findings about visual mental imagery. We focus on visual imagery because that has been the focus of most scientific studies, and thus more is known about such images than images in other modalities (although there has been some intriguing research on motor, auditory, and olfactory imagery).[2]

As we use the term, a "visual mental image" refers to a representation, a physical state that serves to store information; we assume that when such representations are present, they somehow produce the conscious experience of "seeing with the mind's eye." Imagery is an important part of mental life. For example, it plays roles in memory, reasoning, creativity, planning, emotion, and pain control. To be concrete, you should experience the role of imagery in memory retrieval when you answer the following questions: What shape are Mickey Mouse's ears? In which hand does the Statue of Liberty hold the torch? Which is darker green, the skin of an avocado or a lime? In all of these cases, people typically report that they visualize the object or objects when responding. Similarly, if you stub your toe and are in pain, you can visualize yourself walking down a gorgeous beach and putting your toe in the cold water, transforming the pain into a different, less noxious sensation. Many such salubrious functions of imagery have been incorporated into Buddhist practice, and thus there are many potential points of intersection between such practice and scientific studies of the sort we will describe.

Some readers may be confused at this point, not having had the internal sense of using imagery to answer those questions. And in fact it has been known at least since the nineteenth century that introspections about imagery vary and need not directly reveal how the mind works.[3] Some people may report that they are "looking" at the shape of the ears. Other people may not. When there is a difference in reported introspections, we have no way of knowing whether people genuinely differ in their use of images, or whether they simply differ in how they *talk about*, or *report on*, their use of images. This ambiguity is always in place with introspections, so that this is one of the obstacles to making strong claims based on introspective evidence. How, therefore, can we verify what's really going on in the mind? One strategy in the laboratory has been to externalize introspections—to make the subjective objective. This strategy is analogous to using a cloud chamber to track a cosmic ray; you don't actually see the ray, you see the "footprints" it leaves behind. Similarly, we cannot actually see someone else's mental images, but we can see changes in their behavior when they use imagery—and, more recently, we can see changes in their brain.

This chapter has three parts. First it considers the sorts of circumstances in which introspection succeeds in informing us about the nature of imagery. Second, it considers circumstances in which introspection misleads, where at least your initial introspection would lead you to draw incorrect inferences about the mechanisms that underlie mental processing. And third, it considers circumstances in which introspection is silent—it does not tell you anything about the mechanisms that underlie mental processes.

When Introspection Reveals Properties of Mechanisms

Let's briefly review four cases in which introspection succeeds, where it lends insight into the nature of the mechanisms that produce, interpret, and manipulate imagery representations.

MENTAL ROTATION

If you visualize the lowercase letter *p* and then imagine it rotating 180 degrees clockwise, is it another letter? What if you visualize the uppercase version of the letter N and imagine it rotating 90 degrees clockwise—is it another letter? Most people report that they answer these questions by imagining the forms gracefully spinning into the appropriate positions, and that, after the spin, they can "see" the *d* and the *Z*. This introspection turns out to be on target: when the time to respond is recorded, the more you need to rotate the image, the longer it takes. (And so responses for the *N*, which requires a quarter turn, will be faster than responses for the *p*, which needs a half turn.) Roger Shepard and his colleagues report many elegant demonstrations of this "mental rotation" phenomenon.[4] Introspectively it appears that objects are rotating, and sure enough, the greater the imaged rotation, the longer it takes. The introspection does indeed reveal properties of the underlying information processing that actually accomplishes the work of the mind.

MENTAL SCANNING

Let's consider another question that should elicit a specific introspection: Can you say how many windows there are in your living room? We don't actually care about the answer; we care about what you do to try to find the answer. Most people report that they visualize the room and then scan along an image of the room to count the windows, one by one. Our introspections lead us to believe that we can scan across images, and that the further we scan, the longer it takes. And these introspections line up nicely with the results from many experiments.

For example, in one study Stephen Kosslyn and colleagues asked people to memorize a map.[5] The map included seven objects positioned so that there was a different distance between each pair. After the participants became very good at visualizing this map, they were asked to take part in the following task. They first closed their eyes and visualized the map; then they were asked to focus mentally, with their eyes closed, on one location on the map. And then they waited until they heard the name of another object. Half the time this word did in fact name an object that was on the map (such as *tree*), and half the time it did not (for example, *bench*). The participants were to "look," with their eyes closed, at the (imaged) map, and if the second object was on the map they were to scan to it, and push one button when their attention was fixed on it. If they "looked" and could not find the second object, they were to push another button. Both the response and the time to respond were measured. The participants focused on each object equally often at the beginning of the trials, and from that object scanned equally often to each of the other objects. Given the way the seven objects were positioned, they scanned over twenty-one distinct distances.

The results were straightforward. When only the "yes" trials were considered (trials in which participants successfully scanned to the second object from the initial object), the greater the distance between them on the actual map, the longer it took the participants to scan. In fact, an equal increment of time was added for each increment of distance scanned. Just as introspection suggests, when you visualize something, it is as if it were extended in space, and "travel" across the image takes time, just as travel in real space does.

MENTAL ZOOMING

Now try this: first, visualize a butterfly sitting on your index finger, with your arm outstretched. Next, answer this question: What color is its head? In order to answer this question, most people report that they have to "zoom in" to "see" its head. It is as if there were a limit on the image's capacity to show fine detail, so that if the depicted object is too small in the image, some of its details will be obscured (just as they would be in a photo or on a TV screen).

This introspection is also backed up by the results of empirical investigations.[6] For example, in one study the participants visualized an animal at four different apparent sizes (that is, so that it seemed to fill one of four different-size squares. By "size" we didn't mean the size of the actual object, such as a kitten versus a lion, but the size it appeared in the image, as in a photo when the camera is closer or farther from the object). After forming the image, participants were asked about a possible characteristic of the object. Their job was to "look" at the object as depicted in the image. If the object had the characteristic named, they were to find it and then press one button as soon as it was clear in their image. If the object did not have the characteristic, they were to "look" in the relevant location, and once they were sure the characteristic was not present, they were to press another button. For example, with the image of a cat they might have been asked if it had "pointed ears" (a yes response) or "short horns" (a no response). And in fact they required more time to respond when the object was visualized at a smaller size.

Once again the introspection was backed up by data. The smaller a depicted object appears in a mental image, the more difficult it is to "see" its characteristics. In order to "see" the small details, the participants in these studies had to "zoom in" on their images, and the smaller the image, the more zooming was required—and hence the more time was required to respond.

RECOMBINATION

Let's try one more. Visualize an uppercase letter D, and then mentally rotate it 90 degrees counterclockwise so the straight line is on the bottom. Now visualize an uppercase letter J placed under the rotated D so that the top of the J touches the midpoint of the straight side of the D. Does this combined form seem to resemble a familiar object? Can you "see" an umbrella? The first study to use this technique demonstrated that people can, in fact, combine objects depicted in images and notice emergent properties.[7] Introspectively, we seem to be able to manipulate images of objects and then "see" the results— and the data document that we can in fact discover new patterns.

These four examples—mental rotation, scanning, zooming, and recombination—are cases in which introspection succeeds in indicating how information-processing mechanisms operate during imagery. As introspection suggests, at least some of the representations used in visual mental imagery are spatially organized—have a grain, so to speak—and can be manipulated through rotation or recombination to form new objects.

But introspection is not always so effective. It sometimes misleads us. Let's talk about such cases.

When Introspections Mislead

As we have illustrated, laboratory studies have successfully revealed some of the key ways in which visual mental imagery operates. An alternative approach to gaining insight into imagery is to ask people to introspect about their experience. Such reports are not always accurate, however—and they can be outright incorrect. In some cases the initial introspection can be misleading, but the subject can, through training, become sensitive to the difficulty. In other cases the introspection is misleading, but the subject cannot become aware of the problem and training seems not to correct it.

Let's take a look at some examples. First, we'll consider cases in which initial introspections can be misleading but you can learn to notice the difficulty and, at least sometimes, learn to overcome the problem.

MISLEADING INTROSPECTIONS THAT CAN BE DETECTED
Probably the single most misleading aspect of introspection during visual mental imagery is that images seem to be "mental pictures" but they aren't actually pictures, and they do not share many characteristics of pictures. Unlike pictures, objects depicted in mental images: (1) are preinterpreted and thus difficult to reinterpret; (2) have an internal organization that limits how they can be used; and (3) are often incomplete or inaccurate. Let's go through these points one at a time.

Images are preinterpreted. Our mental images are based on memories of objects and events. When we perceived them initially, we interpreted them, organized them, and stored the results. These interpretations and their organization are still present when we later reactivate the memories to create a new image. For example, Daniel Reisberg and his colleagues have shown subjects classic ambiguous figures, such as the famous duck/rabbit optical illusion.[8] When subjects interpret the drawing as a rabbit when they first study it, later they have a very difficult time "seeing" the duck interpretation in their mental image (and vice versa). In perception, we can see either interpretation relatively easily. So mental images are not like pictures in this regard. However, with hints, subjects can be taught how to reinterpret the image—but their success may depend on how good they are at the necessary forms of information processing.[9]

Internal organization. Images have an internal organization that limits how they can be used. Let us give you an example. Visualize the Star of David. Can you "see" two overlapping triangles in that image? That's relatively easy. How about a parallelogram? That is difficult. Why the difference? You stored the star as two overlapping triangles, so it is easy to "see" the triangles, but to see the parallelogram you have to go back over the different units and reorganize the entire figure. The object depicted in your image has an intrinsic organization, and it is difficult to break up that organization. You can become sensitive to this fact, however; then, even when you cannot succeed in reorganizing the image, you can recognize this fact and not be misled into believing that the image is like a static, stable picture.

Incomplete or inaccurate images. Finally, unlike pictures and actual objects, mental images are often incomplete or inaccurate but we don't notice their fragmentary or misleading characteristics. Objects that are depicted in images seem uniformly detailed because we pay attention to the characteristics we include in the image and don't notice what's missing. But there are likely to be gaps in our images nonetheless. For example, visualize a horse. What do its rear knees look like? Most people get this wrong. They think the back legs of a horse look like a human's legs, but in fact they are very different (the "knees" are very high up, and there is another joint beneath that hinges the opposite way as our knees). Their images are inaccurate. Or sometimes they just leave the legs out. The problem is not *just* that the images are inaccurate with regard to the legs, or that the images leave out the legs. The problem is that the images *seem* complete— and that is why introspection is misleading here. You can learn to notice that your images are vague or incomplete, but this is difficult, in part because when you "look," you actually fill in what you are look-ing for—and thus looking for gaps in mental images is a bit like using a flashlight to look for darkness.

In short, our visual mental images are not pictures. But at least in some respects we can learn to recognize key ways in which mental images differ from pictures—and thus overcome the initial impres-sion conveyed by our introspections.

When Introspection Is Silent

We've just discussed situations in which the initial introspection may be misleading but you can learn to notice this—and sometimes even correct your introspection. Now let us consider what happens when introspections are misleading and the subjects do not learn to notice the problem (or at least no researcher has been able to bring them to notice the problem). Let's focus on image generation, which is the act of producing a short-term memory (conscious) image on the basis of information stored in long-term memory. For example, you have stored information in long-term memory about the shape of Mickey Mouse's ears. But until we asked you about their shape, you hadn't generated any image. The image is not what is stored in long-term memory; it is the representation in short-term memory that gives rise to what you experience when you visualize the ears. Image generation is the process of creating an image. For example, visualize the upper-case letters of the alphabet, one by one. Does each letter seem to spring to mind all at once, all in one piece? Introspectively, people re-port that these images seem to appear all at once—just like when let-ters are flashed on a screen. But in fact, the more segments there are in a letter, the longer it takes to form the image (at least if the letters are drawn certain ways).[10] This and other evidence makes it clear that images are created piece by piece, and not (as introspection suggests) all at once.

Why doesn't introspection detect this process in image creation? Each part of the image typically is created in under one-tenth of a sec-ond, and people simply don't notice a sequence of mental events that unfolds that quickly. And by all appearances so far, we cannot be trained to notice such events.

But this is just touching the surface of the limits of introspection. In no case does introspection reveal the nature of the actual mechanisms that make imagery possible. Why is this important? For cognitive scientists and neuroscientists, the taxonomy of mental functions relies on identifying distinct mechanisms (which sometimes correspond to distinct brain systems). And the distinctions between different mental capacities are not in any fashion apparent to introspection.

For example, go back to the three questions we posed at the outset: What shape are Mickey Mouse's ears? In which hand does the Statue of Liberty hold the torch? Which is darker green, the skin of an avocado or a lime? Although it is not evident to introspection, shape imagery (such as the shape of Mickey's ears), spatial imagery (such as the hand holding the torch), and color imagery rely in part on distinct neural systems. Shape processing draws on part of the temporal-lobe complex, spatial processing draws on part of the posterior parietal lobes, and color draws on yet another part of the brain, in the occipital lobes. Yet none of this is in any fashion evident to introspection.

In short, introspection is a very limited tool for understanding mental imagery. In some cases it does reveal properties of underlying mechanisms, but in other cases it misleads—or is simply silent. And here's the crucial point: given just an introspection, how do we know in which category it belongs? Does it reveal properties of mechanisms, mislead us, or is it silent? There's nothing in the introspection itself that signals whether we are catching a glimpse of the levers and pistons underlying processing or are simply noting an illusion—the dust stirred up by workings of the hidden mechanisms within, which does not tell us anything about their nature.

Why Understanding Mechanisms Is Important

Researchers have expended enormous effort over the past decade to demonstrate that certain parts of the brain are used in mental imagery.[11] Why does this matter? Here is one important reason: imagery shares much neural machinery with like-modality perception, and because of this, imagery "inherits" specific characteristics that are used during perception. That is, at least in some cases the characteristics of processing in parts of the brain during perception are also present during imagery. For example, in perception images should not linger; when you move your head and move your eyes, you don't want the images striking your eyes to "smear." So the neurons don't retain the visual input very long. This is good in perception, but it can be a drawback in imagery. The mechanism makes mental images difficult to maintain; they fade quickly.

One reason Buddhist practice is of interest to scientists studying imagery is that the training has been said to result in the ability to maintain images for very long periods of time. If the same areas of the brain used in perception are also used in imagery, this should be extremely difficult—if not impossible. The Buddhist claim seems incompatible with the findings coming from the laboratory, and the Buddhist claim rests entirely on introspection. That is precisely why we needed to walk through a tutorial on what introspection can and cannot do. With that tutorial in view, we now see that we cannot resolve the apparent tension between Buddhist and Western claims until we find a way to get beyond the introspections. In the example of maintaining an image for a long time, it is of course possible that the claims of Western science are in error because (perhaps) the nature of imagery changes with the enormous amount of practice that meditators achieve. But it is also possible that the meditators are mistaken, misled by their introspections. The point is, we cannot resolve this issue through introspection alone; as we have seen, introspections are sometimes revealing and sometimes not.

We do know that experience can fine-tune cognition and the brain in exciting ways, and we may have much to learn from contemplative Buddhists who have refined the art of imagery. Among other questions, we wish to know the limits of the imagery system: in its optimal condition, what can it do? But to understand those limits—and to understand what needs to be changed to improve imagery—we need to understand the mechanisms, and for that we cannot rely solely on introspection. Introspection reveals the *results* of mechanisms at work but not the mechanisms themselves. Although introspections provide important data and must be taken seriously, they must be checked against other forms of evidence if we are to understand the nature and the mechanisms of mental imagery.

Imagery and Visualization

*After the presentations in Part II of the conference, Stephen
Kosslyn and Matthieu Ricard were joined on the stage by
Nancy Kanwisher of the McGovern Institute at MIT;
Daniel Reisberg, professor of psychology at Reed College;
Marlene Behrmann, professor of psychology and neuro-
science at Carnegie Mellon and the University of
Pittsburgh; and Alan Wallace, director of the Santa
Barbara Institute for the Interdisciplinary Study of
Consciousness. The Dalai Lama, we noted jokingly,
would serve on every panel over the course of the week-
end conference.*

ANNE HARRINGTON: I suggest that we start with the most
provocative issue on the table: the Buddhist concept of
pure awareness and luminosity. I was struck, Matthieu,
that in part of your remarks you referred to a concept
that I felt had no real correlate or analogue in the West-

D I A L O G U E

ern tradition. Stephen Kosslyn has said that he has no idea how to handle this fact. Is there any way that brain science or cognitive science could begin to engage with the Buddhist side on this fundamental issue?

ARTHUR ZAJONC: Maybe we should first characterize the phenomenon itself.

MATTHIEU RICARD: Yes, and we can start to do so by offering an example: a mirror has the faculty to reflect images, but there is no image in the mirror itself. Yet without the mirror, you can't have the images. If you can conceive of a mirror without images, you may have an idea of what pure awareness without mental constructs could be. You can't have any thought without this bare cognitive faculty. Usually, when our mind functions, it is in relation to some object: memory, imagination, perception. That's the way we function. We are not used to experiencing this pure awareness that is always there behind the screen of thoughts. We are used to perceiving things—objects, colors, memories, fantasies—but we don't really look at the mind itself. However there could be times, even for an untrained person, when the thought or image is gone and there is a short moment before something else arises, yet you are obviously still aware. You could become more aware of that mere awareness. There could be times that this moment, when it [the mind] is just a mirror, naturally becomes longer. It is a simple awareness, without mental construct, without concept, without imagery, and yet it is definitely there.

STEPHEN KOSSLYN: Matthieu, in your talk you said that when you reach the roof you do not need to put the ladder on your back and carry it with you. I think the implication was that imagery is a method that allows you to reach another place, at which point you abandon imagery. In Western science there is a long history of treating imagery as a primitive form of thought. I just wonder if that is the way it is regarded in Buddhism.

MATTHIEU RICARD: We don't really call it primitive, but we do speak of two stages. We call the first stage the generation, or development, stage, during which you gain the capacity to build up the visualized images. When the mind transformation occurs, you stop clinging to reality as solid or to the "I" as being an entity, and the deluded perceptions are replaced by what we call pure vision—pure in the sense of being undeluded and in harmony with reality. Once this goal is achieved, you are no longer the toy of wild thoughts that keep invading your mind, and you have a clear recognition of that pure awareness. Beyond that point, you do not need to continue to use the ladder that much. Of course, this is the ultimate goal, and until then you need all the tools.

DANIEL REISBERG: Matthieu, if I understand you correctly, you are suggesting that there are certain important privileges that come with this pure awareness. I am reminded of a chapter in the history of twentieth-century physics when Einstein and Heisenberg were writing to each other. Einstein made it clear that to do good science, one had to be able to imagine the things that one was "doing science on." One had to be able to visualize the train moving at light speed with the clock on it, and so on, through the famous thought experiments. In response, Heisenberg thought this was the silliest thing imaginable, and that clearly the only way to do good science was to get past these images and rely on something that I would loosely call pure awareness, although in Heisenberg's case it was clearly a form of awareness that was easily translated into mathematics. But since both these physicists were massively successful in leading us to great discoveries about the deep nature of the world, it makes me think that one might hesitate to identify one or the other of these as the preferred mode. The history of the science seems to suggest that both modes of thinking—one based on imagery and one that held imagery at arm's length—were effective in their own way.

ALAN WALLACE: There is a good analogy here. In physics there is a great deal of research into questions about the nature of space. For example, is there an energy of space? In other words, what kind of energy exists in space when no matter or electromagnetic energy has been introduced into it? In a rather similar fashion, the pure awareness that we speak of in Buddhism is like space. In fact space is a very common metaphor for that experience. At the same time, there are the myriad forms that emerge from space. It's not that one is superior to the other; they are two facets of the same reality. In Buddhism we commonly speak of ultimate and conventional, or relative, reality, but in the final analysis they are of the same nature.

MATTHIEU RICARD: Without the mirror of pure awareness you would never have any mental image.

MARLENE BEHRMANN: The distinction about the sense of a pure awareness suggests some really fundamental differences in the way that Buddhists and cognitive scientists conceptualize imagery. The metaphor of the mirror suggests to me a very passive, reflective process. But in fact there is an assembly, a constructivist approach to visual mental imagery. The components are really built up into some kind of unit. That is one area where I see a difference between the perspective of Buddhist scholars and that of science.

But it permeates other ideas about imagery. Matthieu told us about how imagery is thought to be patterns of light without any associated physical substance—like a rainbow, or a diffusion of light. The perspective of cognitive science has been of images with definitive forms, depictions that have almost physical substance. They aren't pictures, but they are very symbolic isomorphic depictions of the real world. So there seem to be both qualitative and quantitative differences in the way Buddhists think about visual mental imagery and the kinds of representations that Western scientists think exist in the domain of visual imagery.

DANIEL REISBERG: Do Buddhists have an understanding of the concept of individual differences in trainability for visualizing imagery?

DALAI LAMA: It is important to bear in mind the various contexts in which we use the term *imagery*. For example, imagery is thought to be the content of almost all forms of thought that occur naturally, particularly thoughts that follow a sensory experience. If you see something, then you can imagine what you have seen with your eyes closed: that is a thought process that follows after a sensory experience. You don't even have to close your eyes; the same thing happens while you are seeing something but not paying attention to it, instead paying attention only to the mental image. As you do this, eventually, automatically, the active role of eye consciousness diminishes.

However, there is an understanding in the contemplative tradition that the mental imagery that everybody experiences during thought (the technical term is "to generate an image") is meaning-based imagery. It may not necessarily be an image in the sense of a picture but rather some form of concept or construct. One can develop one's capacity to maintain that image and refine it. This is done through meditative practice. Through constant training and familiarity with the image that you conceptualize, you can reach a very high level of clarity, such that the content of that thought is referred to as a form, almost like a visible form. Unlike ordinary material objects that are characterized by shape and color and so on, the content of that thought is not a material object, but it is nevertheless referred to as a mental object that has a form. It is considered a constructed form. There are parallels recognized between this experience of very vivid, clear imagery and the dream state. There is also an understanding that one can further develop one's meditative capacity to a very high level, where that form will take on a qualitatively different nature. For example, if the object of the meditation is a fire, the generated form can burn and one can use it like a real fire.

ALAN WALLACE: This refers to the use of *kasinas* in the Pali tradition. By taking the conceptual quintessence of an element such as fire—it could be another element as well—and generating it meditatively, you can actually project it into the sensory world.

DALAI LAMA: There is a complex understanding of the various levels to which imagery can be trained. The types of practices that Matthieu described are part of a Vajrayana practice referred to as "generation stage."

The discussion of pure awareness triggered a thought for me that is probably more appropriate for a discussion among Buddhists, but I have thought about it for a long time. There are references in Buddhism to phenomena like pure awareness, which is sometimes described as "the clear-light state of mind" or "most subtle state of mind" that becomes manifest at the very moment of death and carries on into the intermediate state after this life. I feel that even in such extremely subtle states of consciousness, the mental state must have some physical base, however subtle it may be. Sometimes there is a tendency among Buddhists to think of these very subtle states of consciousness as if there were no embodiment or material basis for them.

The spirit of my thinking on this is very similar to the basic scientific standpoint: that the brain is the basis for all cognitive events. Without the brain, there could be no function of the mind. So I don't know whether that subtle consciousness could exist independently without a physical base. I don't know. *(laughing)*

ANNE HARRINGTON: Marlene, you had a question about what we should do when the data of brain science and the data of introspection disagree.

MARLENE BEHRMANN: My question is a little more general than that. It has to do with the material basis of visual mental imagery. There appear to be many regions of the brain that are active during the course of perception, and a subset of those same regions are activated during visual mental imagery. It looks as if an elegant property of the brain's design allows you to get two processes out of the same underlying substrate. We don't have a whole lot of brain tissue, and so it makes sense to have both perception and imagery—seeing in the world and seeing in the mind's eye—use the same underlying mechanism.

An empirical question comes to mind. There seems to be a rather small subset of brain regions that are activated in imagery compared with perception. Are advanced contemplative practitioners perhaps recruiting some additional perception areas to subserve this very sophisticated and refined visual mental imagery? It seems an immediately testable hypothesis. If your images get better and better with experience and practice, does that change the brain? Does it result in more of the areas that are normally recruited by perception now being recruited by imagery? What is the substrate?

ALAN WALLACE: For all that Buddhists have been intensely interested in the nature of the mind for 2,500 years, there really is no compelling Buddhist theory of the brain. As you said, brain mechanisms are not revealed by introspection, and I think the Buddhist tradition would probably corroborate that assertion. So the answer is, we don't know.

DALAI LAMA: There is, however, something analogous to what Marlene's question is suggesting. In Buddhist texts, there are primarily two sources. One is known as the Sutra system and one as the Vajrayana system. The Sutra system utilizes the mind only. The Vajrayana system uses not only the mind but also the basis of the mind, which in Buddhist texts is referred to as energy or *prana*.

ALAN WALLACE: This refers to energies within the body that are specifically correlated with mental events. In Vajrayana, or this higher class of practice, you work on two avenues: not only transforming the mind but also explicitly transforming energies in the body. This is said to open up other types of heightened or exceptional awareness.

DALAI LAMA: The contemplative texts of the Sutra system recognize the possibility of cultivating heightened awareness only in relation to visual perception and auditory perception, but not the other senses. There is a similar limitation even in modern technology. You can project images on a television screen, or you can project sounds through radio waves, but you still cannot transport smell and tactile sensations. But in the Vajrayana tradition, given that there is an emphasis on both the mind and also the basis of the mind—the bodily energies for which the primary locus is thought to be in the head—there is an understanding that it is possible for advanced yogis to gain mastery over these physiological elements. Those bodily energies that are normally confined to the function of specific sensory faculties can actually be co-opted or transferred.

For example, a yogi might be able to close his eyes and read a text through his fingers with the sensation of touch. Such claims are made, which suggests the possibility of transferring energies to a different basis.

STEPHEN KOSSLYN: We do know that, if you are blind, your visual cortex is activated when you read Braille. The brain reorganizes itself.

DALAI LAMA: But in this case, it is not through touch that one reads.

ANNE HARRINGTON: Well, there may be more to discuss on that. *(laughter)*

ALAN WALLACE: There is.

MATTHIEU RICARD: It's just the tip of the iceberg. I was puzzling what measurable changes in the brain we would predict for someone who has this faculty of stable and vivid imagery at the time that he is engaged in the practice with stability and clarity. Definitely there should be something stable, or clear, or enhanced in the corresponding part of the brain.

NANCY KANWISHER: I would like to follow up on what Matthieu just said. One of the goals of this conference is to come up with empirically testable hypotheses. I think the one you just suggested is a great idea. If it is really true that after training you can hang on to an image longer, indeed you would expect to be able to pick that up in some way in the brain.

More generally, it seems a whole host of testable hypotheses are floating around here. I thought it would be useful to list some of them. Concerning the training of imagery and of attention, it seems to me that the first important thing to do is to test people behaviorally who have had extensive training, to see if we can pick up behavioral signatures of these claims. Improved mental imagery could take many different forms. People with such training might be able to hold on to images longer, as just mentioned, or they might be able to imagine more items at once. You could test these ideas by measuring the duration and capacity of short-term visual memory. For example, you could present a complicated image with variable numbers of elements in it and test the short-term visual memory of that image a moment later. All these kinds of behavioral measures should be done first, it seems to me, on those with extensive training.

STEPHEN KOSSLYN: When you train your imagery, does it generalize? That is, if you train on images of certain deities, do you later have the same imagery ability with other things you did not train on?

DALAI LAMA: Yes.

MATTHIEU RICARD: Normally it should generalize, because the stability and clarity one achieves are general qualities that can be applied in any circumstances. For instance, when His Holiness gives the initiation of Kalachakra, he has to go through some 720 deities. I personally have seen a retreatant in Tibet, who was also a painter, checking the accuracy of the drawing in some frescoes that depicted over two hundred deities. He was simply looking at them as if he could check them against what he was seeing in his mind. While thus inspecting the frescoes, he would occasionally say, "I think there is a mistake. He's holding the wrong thing in his right hand." It was quite amazing.

So the ability to visualize clearly a deity should generalize, at least to other types of deities. But it may not translate into an increased capacity to do better on all kinds of mental imagery tests, such as rotating objects and others.

STEPHEN KOSSLYN: The reason I ask is because I'm looking for experiments that will disprove my theory. According to my theory, the training should be very specific. The point of contact between your tradition and our tradition is most interesting when we find cases where you have made proposals or claims that contradict what we would predict based on our theories. So maintaining images for twenty minutes or twenty hours is definitely worth testing, but also, more subtly, I would expect such training to be very specific. If you get good at visualizing these deities, it may not affect [your ability to visualize] other deities, let alone a rabbit.

DALAI LAMA: In fact, the text on visualization recommends to practitioners at the beginner's level not to shift focus. Initially you have to stick with cultivating one set of images. But once you have gained a certain mastery, then you have the flexibility to be able to shift and redirect your focus.

ALAN WALLACE: I suspect it is somewhat more complex than this. For example, one of the techniques for mental imagery is to visualize something very simple, like a white pearl of light. Focus on that and do nothing else. You may develop great stability and vividness there. Let's imagine you become adept at focusing on a single pearl of light; then you go to the teacher and he says, "All right. Here are 720 deities. Go for it." I don't think that you will find that you can immediately visualize 720 deities with the same clarity that you could visualize a pearl of light. You will have a head start, but it's a much more complicated feat and it will take you some time to get into that gear.

There are a wide variety of techniques for stabilizing and refining the attention. Some entail a mental image, but another example is focusing on the breath. If you have become very good at focusing on the breath, it doesn't necessarily mean that you will immediately be extremely good at creating mental imagery.

You were asking about pure awareness. Even there, there are relative and ultimate stages of empty awareness. Right now you can be aware that you are aware. Without particularly attending to any of the objects of awareness, you can simply sit there and be immediately aware of being aware. Can you not? You don't have to understand that by inference, do you? What image came to mind when you were simply focusing on being aware of being aware?

Now other thoughts are coming in. Let's do a thought experiment. Imagine you have the knack for that awareness. You know what it's like even though there are a lot of stimuli coming in. Now imagine that we slip you into a sensory deprivation tank and your mind goes very quiet. At least for an interlude, there are no images coming to mind but you haven't fallen asleep or gone dopey. The mind is perfectly clear; it's very stable. Imagine a pure case, where you have no sensory experience of your environment whatsoever but you are not unconscious. That would be a facsimile of pure awareness, where you are aware of being aware. There is something there that is very hard to articulate, but you may be able to imagine it. That is one way to refine the attention to a very high level.

NANCY KANWISHER: But wouldn't you be having thoughts in that situation? Wouldn't you be aware of the thoughts?

ALAN WALLACE: Of course you would.

MARLENE BEHRMANN: Then what's pure about it?

ALAN WALLACE: At the beginning, of course, thoughts are compulsive. They keep on coming just from sheer habit. But as you become more adept at this practice, the density of thoughts starts to thin out. The interludes between thoughts start to expand, and you have longer and longer moments—three seconds, then thirty seconds, then thirty minutes—in which you maintain or even enhance the clarity of awareness. You are vividly aware, but you are vividly aware of not much at all.

STEPHEN KOSSLYN: Matthieu, in your talk you emphasized that meaning was always bound to images. There is a process called "reality monitoring," where people confuse their images with actually having seen something. If I ask you to visualize objects and I also show you objects, and later ask you to select which objects were actually shown versus which ones you visualized, you will make mistakes. It's not surprising, given the information we have on the brain.

At first I worried that if your images got more and more vivid, you would be more prone to mistake having visualized something for having seen something. But if I understood properly, you overcome that problem because you always have the meaning attached to the image, and awareness is improving. Is that correct? Are you able to have increasingly vivid images without confusing them for reality because of the meaning and the awareness attached to the image? Or is there a flip side: do people actually get confused about what they have visualized and what they have seen as they practice more?

MATTHIEU RICARD: I do not have a direct experience of this myself, so I may not be qualified to reply, but for advanced practitioners there are two processes going on at the same time. They increasingly see what we call solid "reality" as being like a dream, an illusion, and at the same time they become increasingly able to visualize mental images vividly. So at some point reality becomes like visions and visions become real.

ALAN WALLACE: I think it could happen.

STEPHEN KOSSLYN: We know that people who have more vivid imagery are more prone to this problem. My question is: Does training with the meaning component help to avoid that problem? Do you become increasingly aware of the distinction between your image and the world? Is that part of what you are training to do?

MATTHIEU RICARD: You try to avoid solidifying the image as something that is really solid, as we normally perceive solid reality. That's why, at the end of every training in visualization, you dissolve the visualization into clear light. This avoids the danger of clinging to it as something solid. That's a very important step. There is a story—I don't know whether it is true or not—of a meditator who was so engaged in visualizing that he did not dissolve it. He was visualizing a deity with a horned animal head, and at one point it is said that the horns were preventing him from getting out of the hermitage. This is an example of a deviation from the visualization practice, because it solidifies the phenomenal world. The goal, rather, is for the visualization to help you to see the whole phenomenal world as an appearance that is void, like a rainbow. The goal is not to cling to realities as being solid.

DANIEL REISBERG: I would like to return to a very important question that His Holiness raised earlier. When the question came up I thought I knew the answer, but as our conversation has progressed, I am less and less certain I know the answer, so let me see if I can voice my confusion. The question was whether there are people who, in some important way, lack the capacity for visualization, whether because of wearing eyeglasses or some such reason. One of the things that psychology has wrestled with for the past hundred years or more is that if you talk to ordinary, untrained people about their experience of imagery, you get an extraordinary diversity of reports. Some people spontaneously report images as if they are looking at very clear, detailed, vivid pictures. People at the other extreme insist that they have never in their lives experienced anything that they could legitimately count as a mental picture.

Psychologists are uncertain what to make of this, and I suspect that you might get several different interpretations from this panel of psychologists. But the observation itself is quite clear-cut. My first take on this was that not being able to visualize would be a significant disadvantage for anyone entering contemplative training, because they would be lacking one of the tools that they need in order to make progress. Then, as the conversation proceeded and you discussed what one achieves after learning to visualize and one starts moving toward these quintessences or pure forms, it sounded like the poor souls who lack visual imagery might actually have a head start. They can proceed immediately to step two and experience these quintessences without the distraction of all the visual forms. I am curious to know whether that latter way of thinking makes sense at all from your understanding of the training, or whether we need more detail about what these individuals lack. I should say, parenthetically, that I am one of those individuals, and so I would like to believe that there are certain advantages associated with this state.

DALAI LAMA: In the training of attention where you are not focusing on a mental image but rather simply focusing right on the very nature of awareness itself, there is a technique for that. As you are abiding in the present, you leave your attention hovering right in the immediacy of the present moment and you block out—with effort—any recollections or thoughts pertaining to the past, and similarly you block out any anticipation or imagining of the future. You remain right there in the moment, abiding in the immediacy of the present without letting your mind fragment either to the past or the future.

This is a strenuous practice. As you venture into this practice, there will be a fair amount of competition for your awareness. You are getting stimuli from the visual, auditory, and other senses. But as you become more adept at this practice, you may have times when your attention is really quite purely focused on just the nature of being aware, right in the moment. Over time you might have a half minute or a minute in which that is all that appears to your mind. It's just awareness itself. The salient features of awareness, which in the Tibetan Buddhist tradition is called *sechen rigpa*, are sheer luminosity, or clarity, and cognizance, or the experience of knowing an event that is going on. For a half minute, or for a minute, you may be so focused on this that only the salient features, the defining characteristics of awareness itself, are manifest. This is something that, at least for a half minute or a minute, could be accessible to an ordinary person. It is not an extremely advanced stage of meditative experience.

DANIEL REISBERG: Surely I am misunderstanding, but it sounds like someone who is dysfunctional as I am, and therefore not distracted by sensory experiences, is already well on the road and therefore should be that much calmer, more centered, and so on. Those in the room who know me know that this is absolutely counterfactual. It makes me think that I do not quite understand what one needs to subtract in order to reach the next stage.

MATTHIEU RICARD: There is an element of clarity that we don't usually have when we simply stay in an ordinary, dull, neutral state without imagery or mental constructs. The answer definitely relates to clarity. When we speak of pure awareness, the element of luminosity or clarity is much increased. There is extreme vividness, open presence, transparence, lucidity. This is not something that we ordinarily experience, because even if you don't notice, there are always a lot of thoughts and perceptions that run in the back of your mind. In a meadow, you may not see the water that is running under the grass, but the water is always there. It is the same with mental chatter that always creates a background noise in your mind. But pure awareness is not like that. It's a sheer clarity, with no element of distraction or torpor or oblivion. That clarity is normally missing in ordinary, dull experience. So there is still some effort to be made.

ANNE HARRINGTON: When monks who enter into a monastery turn out to have poor visualization, what do you do for them?

MATTHIEU RICARD: We are focusing on mental imagery in this session, but it's really only one of many methods. We speak of 84,000 ways of approaching spiritual transformation. Visualization is a very powerful way, but it is certainly not the only one.

ANNE HARRINGTON: The scientists have posed some hypotheses that they would like to see brought into a laboratory, but what would the Buddhists like to see studied? What do you think is important, particularly on the issue of imagery?

ALAN WALLACE: I have a question with regard to the hypothesis that mental images do not happen instantaneously but are generated sequentially. His Holiness already raised the issue of dream imagery. There is also the instance of hypnagogic imagery, which occurs right on the borderline between waking and sleeping. In some cases it may be as vivid as if you are watching a movie at a movie theater. It is radiantly clear and it may be multimodal. In one case of hypnagogic imagery that I had, I was mentally seeing a brook but I was also hearing it, and I could feel the wind blowing through the grass on the side of the brook. It was stable and extremely lucid. That seemed like a preface to the dream state, and dreams, as you know, can go on for forty-five minutes at a time.

Do you think the type of clarity that we have both in hypnagogic imagery and dream imagery is, in principle, inaccessible during the waking state? The corollary question is: When I was seeing that brook, was I generating it drop by drop, frame by frame, or was that not more like visual imagery, like just seeing a brook? From a first-person perspective it certainly seemed like I was mentally seeing a brook.

STEPHEN KOSSLYN: Your intuitions are exactly right. There are many reports of dynamic imagery in some studies, although it is understudied. But it is definitely the case that objects in images move as real objects do. They engage the motor cortex and parts of the cortex that are involved in tracking motion. That has been studied in the scanner. In fact Nancy Kanwisher did some of that implied-motion work.

I think these are all different states, and it is not clear that one is a necessary prerequisite for the other, or even that they overlap much. Spatial imagery, color, and shape draw on different parts of the brain. Dreaming is a sequence of images. You do not maintain just one image. It is fragmented, and the reason for that is that usually your images require action. Our images actually prepare us for moving, and in dreaming, of course, you don't want to move. You have turned off those parts of the brain. Parts of the visual cortex are activated later downstream, but not at the very earliest stage. Dream imagery doesn't look very much like waking imagery on the scanner. It looks like there is a lot of fragmentation and changing.

ALAN WALLACE: The hypothesis from the Buddhist side is that if you train the attention in stability and vividness by using a mental image, when you become adept you can see it mentally with more or less the same degree of clarity and vividness as you would see it with the eyes. True or false, that is the hypothesis. But during a dream state we do see things with the same clarity as if we were seeing with the eyes, at least on some occasions. It seems like there is extraordinary clarity in some dreams. In your understanding, is that degree of clarity of mental images, in principle, inaccessible during the waking state? Buddhism would say no, it's not in principle inaccessible. Do you disagree?

STEPHEN KOSSLYN: First of all, I'm not sure I take the introspection at face value. I suspect people differ markedly in their reports of how clear those images are. Second, even if they do agree, or even if one person is consistent over time, I would want to know which class of introspection those reports fall into, relative to mechanism. Do these very vivid dream images really reflect an underlying state of the mechanism very much like what occurs during vivid perception? That's an empirical question. Finally, even if they did, I would predict that you could not carry the experience over into waking perceptions. There is too much interference when you are awake. The brain is in a different mode. Different transmitter systems are activated. Waking is really quite different from that stage of sleeping.

MATTHIEU RICARD: I think it would be interesting to test the extent to which a clear visualization competes with a clear perception of something that is presented to you. It would seem that, insofar as your visualization is extremely clear—at least for images that are transforming and not just static—you may not be able to see something that actually appears with the same degree of clarity. If you started attending to it, it would be more difficult to maintain the visualization. If you have a very clear visualization, you certainly perceive the whole field before you, with its different colors and shapes, but you are not actually attending to their details and identification. That might be something that could be tested.

MARLENE BEHRMANN: There are very well established laboratory paradigms that lay out the potential interference between imagery and perception. It seems obvious that we should be using these paradigms, which appear to be really robust and scientifically tractable, to evaluate this kind of question. It is a really exciting idea.

NANCY KANWISHER: In one study in my lab, we looked with the scanner at particular parts of the brain that respond to specific types of mental imagery or actual percepts. One region responds very selectively when you look at faces, and another region responds very selectively when you look at scenes. We then had people close their eyes and imagine faces or scenes, and we showed selective activation of the same corresponding brain areas. We looked at the magnitude of the activation in those areas, and it was roughly half as strong in mental imagery as in actual perception. That percentage of activation might be stronger after training.

At this point Anne Harrington, in her role as moderator, changed gears. As in the earlier dialogue session, members of the audience had been invited to write questions on slips of paper, and a small pile of

these questions now sat on the table before Arthur Zajonc, who was
leafing through them. Anne turned and invited Arthur to select some of
the questions for general discussion. He responded by first characteriz-
ing the tenor of the questions as a whole.

ARTHUR ZAJONC: There are quite a number of questions from people who are concerned about the benefits of mental imagery beyond the purely psychological or spiritual benefits. For example,
there's a belief now that certain kinds of mental imagery can have
a benefit for the curing of disease or the control of pain. There are
psychological benefits that might enhance creativity or memory
functions. There is also a question concerning schizophrenia, but
all of these have to do with psychological or even bodily improve-
ments as a result of mental imagery.

MATTHIEU RICARD: I will just describe a few techniques that I use
precisely as applications of mental imagery to alleviate pain or to
increase specific positive emotions like compassion. There is a
well-known type of meditation for pain. If one has a very bad physical pain in one spot, one can imagine, for instance, the image of
a Buddha radiating light at that spot. That light becomes like a
nectar, which is at the same time luminous, warm, and soothing
and which has a pleasing orange color. It completely pervades and
soaks the place where there is pain, then radiates and pervades
your whole body. Doing this again and again is known to help to
alleviate the feeling of pain. It's regularly used by meditators who
have acute physical pain, and they find it very beneficial.

A way to use mental imagery to enhance one's positive emotions is with the meditation we call "the exchange of happiness
and suffering." You use your breathing, which is the most natural
function we have. When you breathe in, you imagine that you are
gathering all the suffering and pain of all sentient beings like a
dark cloud. You visualize that you are drawing it in like a cloud of
smoke and absorbing it into your heart, which you visualize as a
bright mass of white light. As the black cloud completely dissolves
into that light, you visualize that all the sufferings of sentient be-

ings are being dissolved. Then, as you breathe out, you breathe all your loving kindness, compassion, and whatever happiness you might have to all sentient beings. It's not like you cut a piece of cake and distribute it; rather, every sentient being gets it whole. You do this again and again, riding on the breath, doing it just as naturally as you breathe in and out. It is a visualization that completely transforms your mind in terms of the concepts of happiness, suffering, and generating compassion. Because it's linked with the breath, it really helps transform your mind toward compassion.

This is an amplification of mental imagery, and there are all sorts of variations. You might think of your body transforming into whatever other beings might need. For those who need food, you become food. For those who need clothes to protect them from the cold, you become the clothes. Everywhere in the world, whatever is needed, your body transforms. This is mental imagery, but the goal is to really open your mind and increase your loving kindness and compassion. We find many uses of mental imagery to actually effect the transformation that we are looking for.

ARTHUR ZAJONC: I think this next question I have was directed toward the scientists. The Buddhists may present certain practices and, based on their own experience, believe that these are of benefit in relieving pain or even perhaps in helping with certain kinds of illnesses. Is there space within your understanding of the mind and its relationship to the body to accommodate this?

STEPHEN KOSSLYN: There is something I call the reality simulation principle, which is based on the idea that so much neural real estate is shared by imagery and perception. It says that most effects that can occur by interacting with an object in the world can be mimicked by interacting with objects and mental images. We know that by looking at an object you can remember it better than when you just hear its word. If you visualize the object, you will remember it about twice as well as you do just looking at the word. These studies go back hundreds of years. You can double your memory ability by using imagery. Mental practice has a more complicated literature, but in a meta-analysis, the studies suggest that by rehearsing certain behaviors, you will actually get better at doing those behaviors.

MATTHIEU RICARD: Aren't there studies on pain control that show that, of all the distractions that have been tried, mental images are the most efficient?

STEPHEN KOSSLYN: That's correct. There have been meta-analyses of all the studies on psychologically based pain control, and mental imagery is the best in every case.

DANIEL REISBERG: There is ample research literature on the role of visualization techniques in creative problem solving. The literature is quite striking in that there are things that you can do with imagery and things that you cannot. For example, some very interesting studies of practicing professional architects look at what sorts of problems they solve by visualizing the plan they are trying to build, without picking up a pencil, and what other kinds of problems seem to demand that they pick up a pencil and start drawing. It's not a simple equation that imagery helps creativity. It does in some very important regards, but not in all regards.

ALAN WALLACE: I would like to add a corollary to the practice of "the exchange of happiness and suffering" that Matthieu described. His Holiness was asked yesterday how we can possibly experience compassion for a person who engages in evil, especially if this very harmful behavior is directed toward ourselves. His Holiness addressed this by pointing out that the person who engages in evil is himself or herself subject to mental afflictions—to hatred, delusion, greed, and so forth. It is because the person is dominated by mental afflictions that this very harmful behavior is expressed. An appropriate visualization practice would be to attend to such a person and imagine that person free of those mental afflictions, like a doctor imagining a patient without the illness. One then wishes, "May it be so." This may then be followed by the practice that Matthieu just described. But it is important to be able to differentiate between the person and the evil that a person is immersed in as a result of mental afflictions. This is a rather demanding challenge to imagination as well.

ANNE HARRINGTON: Arthur, do you want to put a few more questions on table?

ARTHUR ZAJONC: Certainly. Here's another one. It's kind of a challenge. Imagine that brain imaging studies found that brain activation in trained practitioners showed precisely the same pattern of quickly fading brain activity following imagery as in untrained people. In other words, there was no difference. If it actually turned out that trained subjects were just like everybody else, even though in self-reports they claimed that they could visualize for twenty-four hours or even twenty minutes, would this cause you to question the reality of sustained images?

NANCY KANWISHER: I would say first that failing to see a difference in a brain imaging study is not very informative, and it wouldn't worry me. It is the most common outcome of any brain imaging study. There are many ways to not see a difference in the brain that is actually there. This is a picky point; I am simply pointing out that if you don't get a difference, that's not worrisome. However, if you did the behavioral experiments that we were starting to sketch before and you still did not see differences, then I would start to worry.

ARTHUR ZAJONC: What's the difference? Why is there more reliability in the behavioral experiments?

NANCY KANWISHER: Because the claims are behavioral: that mental-imagery ability is improving. The relationship of that improvement to the brain is unknown. But if mental-imagery ability is improving, let's see it with a behavioral experiment that directly tests the claim.

MARLENE BEHRMANN: From the empirical side of the practitioner's experience, we should not forget that the goal of mental imagery is to help you have a different perception of the phenomenal world and of the way the mind works, eventually getting some kind of inner freedom from obscuring emotions. If in practice you are actually progressing in that, and you see after some months or years that it's true—you are no longer so prone to anger, jealousy, and so forth—from that perspective, the difference would be quite obvious to you yourself in your behavior. You would not worry too much if you didn't see it in brain studies.

ALAN WALLACE: The training of attention is not done in total isolation, as if it were some utterly independent function of the mind. The training of attention takes place along with, and is deeply enmeshed with, training in developing greater emotional balance: less anger; less emotional oscillation between craving and hostility, excessive hope and fear, elation and depression. In this overall balancing of the mind there is attentional balance, emotional balance, and also cognitive balance. The training in what I call cognitive balance—honing mindfulness and clarity of attention so that you are seeing accurately what is there—is really a prerequisite for the more advanced training in visualization in the generation stage of Vajrayana practice.

MARLENE BEHRMANN: Returning to the point that Nancy Kanwisher made about brain activity compared with differences in behavioral performance, there is still the claim that's made by contemplative virtuosos that imagery emerges like a fish out of water, all of a piece. We haven't really delved into this, and it seems really perplexing from a Western scientific perspective. It seems to me that that is an immediately testable hypothesis. Without going into some of these much more murky issues about advanced thought and pure awareness, it's something that lends itself very immediately and obviously to laboratory testing.

MATTHIEU RICARD: That's true. This is something that we find again and again in the description of contemplative practice, especially in advanced stages of meditation. But I wish I could see those visualizations like a fish leaping out of water, so I'm not the right subject for that.

DALAI LAMA: Insofar as the yogi himself or herself is concerned, if he or she experiences a marked reduction in the occurrence of afflictive emotions, whether that can be detected through scientific method is really irrelevant. But at the same time, talking about this triggered a question for me based on current neuroscientific understanding. There seems to be a markedly different location of brain activity for positive emotions, like compassion, and negative emotions, like fear, anger, or hostility. I would be interested to see if there is any difference that one can detect between higher cognitive states of afflictions. For example, from the Buddhist point of view an extreme grasping at self-centeredness or reification of self is thought to be a highly cognitive affliction. It is not an impulsive or reactive emotion like anger or hostility, but grasping too much at the existence of self as core is seen as a cognitive affliction. I wonder whether one could detect any changes in brain activity between that and the directly opposite state of mind, which is believing in the absence of such an intrinsically real self. I would speculate that probably the activation occurs at the same place.

ANNE HARRINGTON: We will have more to say about all this in our session on emotion tomorrow, so perhaps it would be best to hold further discussion of this until then. We now have time for just one more question.

ARTHUR ZAJONC: This question is directed to the scientists. The questioner asks: "Do the scientists have plans to conduct experiments on monks and other practitioners in meditation to determine whether they are in fact better able to hold mental images in their heads? If in fact it proves true, how will it change your theory?" Having put this question on the table, I would like to take the liberty of elaborating on it a little bit, as a physicist. There are certain aspects of theory that are relatively easy to change, and there are others that are grounded in very deep principles, such as conservation laws. It would do real violence to the theory to make changes at that level. The data have to be very compelling. What would it mean for your theories if some of these experiments were to contradict them? At what level would the transformation of theory need to be undertaken?

STEPHEN KOSSLYN: The answer to the first part is definitely yes. We have already started collaborating with and testing monks, but it's proving difficult to find practitioners who have the right sort of expertise in imagery. It is not quite as easy as we thought it was going to be. We have already set up the experiments that test the ability to hold on to images over time, and how vivid they are, and the effects of different kinds of emotions on how easily you can hold images. Those experiments are ready to go. We're waiting to see if we can find someone who will collaborate on that.

Arthur's question really depends on how the results come out and, furthermore, what they reflect. Once we had a behavioral result, we would then scan the monks during that behavior, if they agree, with the object of trying to discover exactly what the mechanism is doing differently. It would really depend. My own view is, if there comes a point where a theory needs to be patched up too much, you just give up and start over again. This might end up being such a case. We have to wait and see how it comes out. It could really lead to something quite new, at least for science.

IV

EMOTION

An Abhidharmic View of Emotional Pathologies and Their Remedies

It is often assumed that one of the strengths of Buddhism is its ability to provide ideas and practices relevant to the emotional domain. After all, Buddhism aims at developing wholesome states of mind, such as equanimity and compassion, and at freeing the mind from negative ones, like grasping and anger. So it seems quite reasonable to assume that the tradition has developed rich ways of understanding the affective domain. This assumption is reflected in a number of contemporary works examining the crossovers between Buddhism and Western psychology. But how warranted is the assumption?

I will respond by providing a brief overview of some of the Buddhist conceptualizations of the affective domain and offer a critical examination of those views, without assuming that Buddhist terms can be easily translated into our usual mental vocabulary. After introducing a more general Buddhist view of the mind and discussing its relevance to understanding the affects, I will lay out some of the Buddhist views of the mind as they are found in the Abhidharma tradition in particular, and discuss the various mental typologies contained in this rich body of texts, underlining their relevance to our modern understanding of emotions. Finally, I will discuss some of the Buddhist techniques that are most relevant to the transformation of the affective life, and raise some questions relevant to our dialogue.

My presentation differs from those of my colleagues in that, rather than examining empirical findings, I essentially follow a philosophical method. I focus on the analysis of Buddhist concepts, which I try to present in their own terms as much as is possible, instead of assuming the unconditional validity of the modern scientific and philosophical perspectives. I believe that it is important that Buddhist ideas about the mind, however alien they may first seem, be taken seriously in such a dialogue. Otherwise the discussion may well remain one-sided, with scientists taking Buddhist practices as their objects and seeing Buddhist practitioners as their guinea pigs rather than as prospective colleagues.

Emotions and Typologies

So what are some of the Buddhist ideas of emotions? Let me start with a shocker: there are no Buddhist conceptions of emotion in the proper sense of the term. By this statement I do not mean to deny that Buddhism has a lot to say about the affective life, but I do mean to say that the concept of emotion as we know it plays practically no role in the traditional Indian and Tibetan Buddhist discussions of the mind. There is no term in the traditional Buddhist vocabulary that resembles our notion of emotion, and our concept of emotion is not recognized indirectly either. This may surprise, since the notion of emotion seems so self-evident and so basic to our modern ways of understanding ourselves. We may imagine people who do not have exactly the same emotional vocabulary as we do, but it seems hard to conceive of people who do not understand a concept as fundamental as that of emotion. And yet this seems to be the case for Buddhists, for in traditional Indian and Tibetan Buddhist texts there does not seem to be any word that even comes close to our concept of emotion.

This surprising and even shocking absence is certainly intriguing. It shows that the idea of emotion, which seems self-evident, is not. Mental concepts, even the ones such as emotion that may seem obvious, are not self-standing. They exist and make sense only within the confines of a mental typology in which they are distinguished from other categories. In the West, perhaps the most famous such typology is Plato's threefold division of the soul: "One part, we say, is that with which a man learns, one is that with which he feels anger. But the third part . . . we called it the appetitive part because of the intensity of its appetites concerned with food, drink, and love and their accompaniments."[1] For Plato, the mind is composed of three parts: reason, the passions, and the appetites. The first helps humans to assess situations and make judgments about what is useful, good, et cetera. But the mind is also often directed by other forces, which Plato describes as the appetites (desire for food) and *thumos*, the principle of high-spiritedness (as when we feel anger), which came to be interpreted as passion and later as emotion. It is only in opposition to each other that these parts of the mind make sense. Hence, a concept such as emotion makes sense only within the confines of a mental typology that is embedded within a broader cultural context and changes historically.

The absence of the concept of emotion in the Buddhist vocabulary also suggests that Buddhists must have a very different way of understanding the mind. So what is this way? What does a typical Buddhist mental typology look like? To answer these questions, I will draw from one of the most ancient Buddhist traditions, the Abhidharma. But before I do so, let me insist that this is not *the* Buddhist view of the mind but just *a* Buddhist view. Buddhism is a complex and multifaceted tradition that has many mental typologies. The view that I present here is only one of the several Buddhist views, though a very widely accepted one.

The Abhidharma Tradition

The Abhidharma is one of the oldest Buddhist textual traditions. It can be traced back to the first centuries after the Buddha (566–483 BCE), when the inspirational teachings of the founder as found in the sutras became systematized. First elaborated as lists,[2] the Abhidharma contains the earlier texts in which Buddhist concepts were developed. As such, it has been the source of most philosophical developments in Indian Buddhism. But the Abhidharma is not limited to this role as source of Buddhist philosophical development. At least until the seventh or eighth century CE, it remained a vital focus of Buddhist thinking and kept evolving. Hence, the Abhidharma is a very large tradition whose diversity we cannot even start to approach. In this discussion, I will simplify greatly my task and consider only a few among the numerous texts of this extremely rich and profuse tradition, focusing mostly, though not solely, on the works of Asaṇga and Vasubandhu, two Indian thinkers from the fourth or fifth century CE. I will also consider at times the Theravada Abhidharma, which received its canonical formulation around the same time through Buddhaghosa's works.[3] All these figures lived during the period often described as the golden age of Buddhist thought in India, when the Abhidharmic tradition was at its apex. In analyzing their views, I will also resist offering a more fine-grained analysis of their conflicting opinions to focus on the general points on which they mostly agree.

The object of the Abhidharma is to analyze the realm of sentient experience and the world given in such experience, in its components, in a language that avoids the postulation of a unified subject. This analysis concerns the whole range of phenomena, from material phenomena to nirvana. For example, there are elaborate discussions of the four primary and four secondary elements that make matter.[4] There are also lengthy treatments of the nature, scope, and types of soteriological practices prescribed by the Buddhist tradition, a central focus of the Abhidharma. But a large part of the Abhidharmic discourse focuses on the analysis of the mental and its different components. Hence, it is often called, somewhat misleadingly, "Buddhist psychology."[5] It is on this part of the Abhidharma that I focus.

In considering experience, the Abhidharma proceeds in a rather characteristic way that may be disconcerting for newcomers but that reflects its historical origin. For each type of phenomenon considered, the Abhidharma analyzes it into its basic elements (dharma), lists these elements, and groups them into the appropriate categories. Thus the study of the Abhidharma often revolves around the consideration of series of extended lists. This is in fact how the Abhidharma started, as mnemotechnic lists of elements abstracted from the Buddha's discourses. I am sure you are familiar with the joke, "Buddhists don't have God, but they sure do have lists!" This is truer of the Abhidharma than of any other Buddhist tradition. So be forewarned.

In elaborating these lists of components of experience and the world given in experience, the Abhidharma is not just reenacting its origin but also embodying one of the central tenets of Buddhist philosophy, the twin ideas of nonsubstantiality and dependent origination. According to this philosophy, the phenomena given in experiences are not unitary and stable substances but complex and fleeting formations of basic elements whose arousal is dependent on complex causal nexuses. This is particularly true of the person, who is not a substantial self but a construct coming to be, dependent on complex configurations of mental and material components (the aggregates). This analysis is not, however, just limited to the person but is applied to other objects. All larger things are analyzed as being composed of more basic elements. Moreover, and this is very important, these basic elements should be thought of not as reified or stable entities but as dynamically related momentary events instantaneously coming into and going out of existence. Thus, when the Abhidharma analyzes matter as being made up of basic components, it thinks of those components less as stable particles, little grains of matter, than as fleeting material events coming and going out of existence and dependent on causes and conditions. Similarly, the mind is analyzed into its basic components, the basic types of events that make up the complex phenomenon we call "mind."

Finally, this Abhidharmic analysis is not just philosophical. It has practical import as well. Its aim is to support the soteriological practices that the tradition recommends. The lists of material and mental events are used by practitioners to inform and enhance their practices. For example, the list of mental factors we will examine shortly is a precious help for various types of meditation, providing a clear idea of which factors need to be developed and which are to be eliminated. In this way, the Abhidharma does not simply function as the source of Buddhist philosophy but also informs and supports the practices central to the tradition, as we will see later.

Abhidharmic Views of Mind

In talking about mind, it is important to understand what one means, for this term is far from unambiguous. According to the Abhidharma, mind is not a brain structure or a mechanism for treating information. It is also not an organ working for a self. Rather, mind is conceived as a complex cognitive process consisting of a succession of related momentary mental states. These states are at least in principle phenomenologically available; that is, they can be observed by turning inward and observing the way in which we feel, perceive, think, remember, and so on. When we do this, we notice a variety of states of awareness, and we also notice that these states change rapidly. It is these mental states arising in quick succession that the Abhidharma tradition identifies as being the basic elements of mind.

It should be clear from this preliminary characterization that in elaborating a theory of the mind the Abhidharma primarily relies on what we would call a first-person approach. It is by looking inward that we gain an understanding of the mind, not by studying it as an object and attending to its external manifestations. This approach of the Abhidharma is not unlike that of many Western thinkers, such as Franz Brentano, William James, and Edmund Husserl, who agree that the study of the mind must be based on the observation of internal mental states. This approach is well captured by James's famous claim that, in the study of the mind, "Introspective Observation is that we have to rely on first and foremost and always."[6]

As James himself recognized, however, the observation of the mind, which seems to make sense intuitively, is not a simple affair and raises numerous questions. What does it mean to observe the mind? Who observes? What is being observed? Is the observation direct or mediated? Besides these difficult epistemological points, there are also questions about the reliability of observation. We are all able to certain degrees to observe our mind, but it is clear that our capacities to do so differ. If this is so, whose observations are to be considered reliable? This question is significant for the Abhidharmists, who may include in their data not just ordinary intuitions but also the observations of trained meditators. There is obviously an important difference in these observations, though the degree to which meditative experience is relevant to Buddhist theories of the mind is not always obvious, as we will see shortly.

The comparison between the Abhidharma and the views of James, the Harvard philosopher, goes further than their reliance on an introspective method. They also share some substantive similarities, the most important of which is perhaps the idea of the stream of consciousness. In the Abhidharma, mental states do not arise in isolation from each other. Rather, each state rises out of preceding moments and gives rise to further moments, thus forming a mental stream or continuum *(santāna, rgyud)*, much like James's stream of thought.[7] The metaphor of the stream is also found in the Buddhist tradition, where the Buddha is portrayed as saying, "The river never stops: there is no moment, no minute, no hour when the river stops: in the same way, the flux of thought."[8]

Unsurprisingly, there are also some distinctions to be made between James and the Abhidharma, differences that will take us into the heart of our topic. A first distinction of some interest to modern research is the question of whether mental states arise in continuity or not. James's view is well known. For him, "consciousness does not appear to itself chopped up in bits."[9] The content of consciousness might be changing, but we move smoothly from one state to another without any apparent break. The Abhidharma disagrees, arguing that although the mind is rapidly changing, the transformations are discontinuous. It is only to the untrained observer that the mind appears to flow continuously. A deeper observation reveals, claims the Abhidharmist, that the stream of consciousness is made of moments of awareness, moments that can be individuated.

Several Abhidharma texts even offer measurements of this moment, measurements that one would expect to be based on empirical observation. But as we noted earlier, such claims are rarely unproblematic, and this is clearly the case here, for different Abhidharma traditions make claims that are, at times, strikingly at odds with each other. For example, the *Mahāvibhāṣā*, an important text from the first centuries of the common era, states that there are 120 basic moments in an instant. The text further illustrates the duration of an instant by equating it to the time needed by an average spinner to grab a thread. Not at all, argues another text; this is too coarse. A moment is the sixty-fourth part of the time necessary to click one's fingers or blink an eye.[10] Although these measurements differ, one could still argue that, given the imprecision of premodern time measurement, there is a rough agreement between these accounts, which present a moment of awareness as lasting for about one-hundredth of a second. This is significantly faster than the transformation of brain states as understood by modern neurology. But consider this other claim made by a Theravada Abhidharma text, that "in the time it takes for lightning to flash or the eyes to blink, billions of mind-moments can elapse."[11] The time scale in this account, which is standard in the Theravada tradition, is faster by many orders of magnitude.

This dramatic discrepancy alerts us to some of the difficulties with accounts based on observation, for whom are we to believe? Which tradition should we rely on? Moreover, we cannot but wonder about the sources of these differences. Do they derive from the observations of meditators, or are they the results of theoretical elaborations? It is hard to come to a definitive conclusion in the face of such large differences, but it seems to me that what we have here are not just empirical observations but largely theoretical discussions, perhaps supplemented by observational reports. Hence, we should be cautious in assuming that these texts reflect empirical findings. Although some may, they are mostly theoretical elaborations that cannot be taken at their face value. Finally, another Abhidharma text seems to further muddy the waters by claiming that the measure of a moment is beyond the understanding of ordinary beings. Only enlightened beings can measure the duration of a moment.[12] Thus it is not surprising that we are left wondering.

Another significant—and for our purpose, more important—difference between James and the Abhidharma is the way the latter conceives of the cognitive functions of mental states. In the Abhidharma, as for James, mental states are intentional; that is, they bear on objects that appear to exist independently of the mental states. But this intentionality is analyzed in different ways. This is where the Abhidharma offers a schema that is to my knowledge quite unique. Considering it will give us the opportunity to understand the ways in which this tradition conceives affective states.

Each mental state, I said, bears on an object. This cognitive relation is described by the Abhidharma as having two aspects: the primary factor of awareness (*citta, gtso sems*), whose function is to be aware of the object, and mental factors (*caitesika, sems byung*) whose function is to qualify this awareness and determine the qualitative nature of the awareness as pleasant or unpleasant, focused or unfocused, calm or agitated, positive or negative, and so on. Vasubandhu in his commentary on his own summary of the Abhidharma explains: "Cognition or awareness apprehends the thing itself, and just that; mental factors or *dharmas* associated with cognition, such as sensation, et cetera, apprehend special characteristics, special conditions."[13]

The basic insight behind this unusual view is that mental states have two types of cognitive functions. The mental state is aware of an object. For example, the sense of smell is aware of a sweet object. But mental states are not just states of awareness. They are not passive mirrors in which objects are reflected. Rather, they actively engage their objects, apprehending them as pleasant or unpleasant, approaching them with a particular intention, et cetera. In my example, my olfactive cognition of a sweet object is not just aware of the sweet taste; it also apprehends the object as pleasant, distinguishes certain qualities, such as its texture, and categorizes the object as being my favorite Swiss chocolate. This characterization of the object is the function of mental factors. The study of these mental factors is important for our purpose, for it is among them that we will find the states we describe as emotions. But before going into this, let us get a firmer grip on these notions by following the standard Abhidharmic procedure—that is, by examining some of the lists through which these concepts are elaborated.

Awareness

Every mental state, I said, is composed of a primary factor of awareness and several mental factors. The primary factor of awareness, which is also described as *vijñāna (rnam shes)*, a term often translated as consciousness or cognitive awareness, is the aspect of the mental state that is aware of the object. It is the very activity of cognizing the object, not an instrument in the service of an agent, the nonexistent self. This awareness merely discerns the object, as in my example where I apprehend the taste of what turns out to be my favorite Swiss chocolate. Hence, Vasubandhu speaks of awareness as the "bare apprehension of each object."[14]

In most Abhidharmic texts, there are six types of awareness: five born from the five physical senses (sight, hearing, smell, taste, and touch) and mental cognition. Each type of sensory cognition is produced in dependence on a sensory basis, one of the five physical senses, and an object. This awareness arises momentarily and ceases immediately, to be replaced by another moment of awareness, and so on. The sixth type of awareness is mental. It is considered by the Abhidharma as a sense, like the five physical senses, though there are disagreements about its basis.[15]

Some Abhidharma texts, such as Asaçga's, argue that these six types of consciousness do not exhaust all the possible forms of awareness. To this list, he adds two types of awareness: the store-consciousness *(ālaya-vijñāna, kun gzhi rnam shes)* and afflictive mentation *(kliṣṭa-manas, nyon yid)*.[16] The idea of a store-consciousness is based on a distinction between the six types of awareness, which are described as manifest cognitive awareness *(pravṛtti-vijñāna, 'jug shes)*, and a more continuous and less manifest form of awareness, the store-consciousness. This consciousness contains all the basic habits, tendencies, propensities, and latent karma accumulated by the individual. It is also a different kind of awareness in that it is subliminal and thus usually remains unnoticed. It is only in special circumstances, such as fainting, that its presence can be noticed or at least inferred.

This consciousness is mistaken by the afflictive mentation as being a self, thus forming the core of our innate sense of self. From a Buddhist point of view, however, this sense is mistaken. It is imposing a unity where there is just a multiplicity of interrelated physical and mental events. Hence, the sense of control that this cognitive core of the person contains is largely mistaken. There is really nobody in charge of the physical or mental processes, which arise according to their own causes and conditions, not following our whims. The mind is ruled not by a central unit but by competing factors whose strength varies according to circumstances.

Thus, Asaçga posits as many as eight types of consciousness. Although exploring the final two types of awareness is outside of our purview, these are important topics, particularly within the context of a dialogue between Buddhism and cognitive sciences.[17] It is true that these notions are associated with a particular school of Buddhist thought, the Yogācāra, which view does not need to detain us here, and that some of the details associated with these concepts may be questionable. Nevertheless, I would insist that the notions about these two types of awareness contain some important insights without which there is no complete understanding of the depth of Buddhist views of the mind.

Mental Factors

Mental states are not, however, just states of awareness. They also actively engage their objects, qualifying them as pleasant or unpleasant, approaching them with a particular attitude, and so on. This engagement is accomplished by mental factors, which are the aspects of the mental state that characterize the object of awareness. To put it otherwise, whereas consciousness makes known the mere presence of the object, mental factors make known the particulars of the content of the awareness, defining the characteristics and special conditions of its object. They qualify the apprehension of the object as being pleasant or unpleasant, attentive or distracted, peaceful or agitated, et cetera.

The translation of the term for these elements of the mind as "factors" is meant to capture the range of meanings that the Abhidharma associates with this term, for the relation between cognitive awareness and mental factors is complex. At times the Abhidharma envisages this relation diachronically, as being causal and functional: factors cause the mind to apprehend objects in particular ways. At other times, however, the Abhidharma seems to emphasize a synchronic perspective, in which cognitive awareness and mental factors coexist and cooperate to carry out the same cognitive task.[18]

In accordance with its procedure, the Abhidharma studies mental factors by listing them, establishing the ways in which they arise and cease, and grouping them in the appropriate categories. Each Abhidharma tradition has a slightly different list. Here I will follow a list of fifty-one mental factors distributed in six groups:[19]

five omnipresent factors
five determining factors
four variable factors
eleven virtuous factors

six root afflictions
twenty branch afflictions.

The nature of this complex typology is clearer when one realizes that these six groups can be further reduced to three. The first three groups contain all the neutral factors. They are the factors that can be present in any mental state, whether positive or negative, and thus these factors are neither positive or negative in and of themselves. Quite different are the next two groups, the virtuous factors and the afflictions. These factors are ethically determined. Their very presence marks the mental state as virtuous or afflictive. The list of factors then becomes:

fourteen neutral factors (five omnipresent, five determining, and
    four variable factors)
eleven virtuous factors
twenty-six afflictions (six root and twenty branch afflictions).

As should be clear from this way of grouping the factors, the Abhidharma typology is explicitly ethical. It is organized around the opposition between virtuous and afflictive factors. It is in the ethically determined categories that one finds the greatest number of factors (thirty-seven), the remaining fourteen being the common cognitive basis of the ethically determined factors.

Although this is not the place to explore the multiple dimensions of ethics in the Buddhist tradition, I do need to say a few words about the ethical character of mental states. For example, how is this ethical character determined? To answer this question, it may be relevant to make a distinction between ethics and morality, a distinction that goes back to Hegel and has been developed by contemporary thinkers such as Paul Ricoeur.[20] Put briefly, the distinction between ethics and morality marks two domains of ethical life. Morality is the more limited domain of rules and injunctions, whereas ethics concerns the more global dimensions of a life lived in accordance with the practice of virtues and oriented toward the good.

This distinction helps us to understand the ethical nature of the

Abhidharma mental typology. Mental states can be assessed morally—that is, from the point of view of whether they are virtuous or nonvirtuous. From this moral perspective, the positive or negative valence of mental states is appraised in terms of karma. Virtuous mental states lead to positive karmic results in this and in future lives, whereas nonvirtuous ones lead to negative results. This distinction certainly exists in the Abhidharma tradition, where one finds discussions of the nature of mental states in terms of karmic results. This is not, however, the main way in which the nature of mental factors is discussed. The distinction I made between virtuous and afflictive factors is different from that between virtuous and nonvirtuous states, though they obviously overlap. Virtuous mental factors are not just ethically positive, they are also morally so. But afflictive factors need not be nonvirtuous. This is true, for example, of the grasping to self, which is morally neutral (it formally violates no rule or injunction) though it is ethically afflictive (it undermines one's capacity to live a virtuous life).

But what, then, do we mean by ethically virtuous or afflictive? The distinction is based on a eudaemonist view of human beings as being first and foremost concerned with happiness, here understood not as pleasure but as well-being and flourishing. Well-being is not easy to attain, since we ordinarily find it hard to sustain happiness. We tend to fall prey to certain tendencies or afflictions, such as self-grasping, attachment, and aversion, that lead us to dissatisfaction and restlessness. These factors are afflictions in that we do not choose to entertain them but they are deeply engrained in us and lead us to suffering. The goal of Buddhist practice is to free ourselves from these inner compulsions so that we may lead a good life through the development of virtues such as detachment and compassion. It is in this sense that the Abhidharma distinguishes between virtuous and afflictive factors.

The virtuous factors are the ones that lead to long-lasting peace and happiness. They are the excellencies, such as compassion and detachment, that are conducive to and constitute the good. These attitudes are positive in that they do not compel us toward attitudes that lead to suffering. They leave us undisturbed, open to encountering reality with a more relaxed and freer outlook. The afflictive factors, on the other hand, disturb the mind, creating frustration, restlessness, and the like. They are the main obstacles to the life of the good as understood by the Buddhist tradition. Asaçga defines afflictions in this way: "The characteristic of affliction is that, when it arises, it has the characteristic of disturbance and renders the mind and the body troubled."[21] It is in this ethical way that the typology of the Abhidharma has to be understood. It offers an analysis of the internal conditions necessary to living a good life by distinguishing the ethically virtuous factors from the afflictive ones.

Some Cognitive and Affective Functions of Mental Factors

Now that we have a handle on the main lines of the Abhidharmic typology, let us focus on the mental factors, delineating some of their cognitive and affective functions. This will allow us to understand the Abhidharma's discussion of the affective domain and its place within the overall mental landscape. First, let us consider the neutral factors. Here is the list:

five omnipresent factors: feeling, discernment, intention, attention, contact
five determining factors: aspiration, appreciation, mindfulness, concentration, intelligence
four variable factors: sleep, regret, investigation, analysis.[22]

These are the factors that are neutral in character in that they can occur in ethically positive, negative, or neutral states. There is obviously a lot to say about this list, which at times seems to involve disparate elements. Here I will have to limit myself to a few remarks.

Among these fourteen factors, the first five are described as omnipresent because they are present in every mental state. Even in a subliminal state such as the store-consciousness, these five factors are present. The other nine factors are not necessary for the performance of the most minimal cognitive task (the apprehension of an object, however dimly and indistinctly). Hence, they are not present in all mental states, only in some.

One striking feature of this list is the preeminent place of feeling *(vedanā, tshor ba)* as the first of the factors. On the one hand, this emphasis reflects the fundamental outlook of the tradition, which views humans as being first and foremost sentient. As such, they are not distinct from other types of beings, such as animals, though they obviously have different abilities. In the Buddhist tradition, all beings are first sentient in that happiness and suffering (in the extended sense of the terms) are for them the foremost issues. On the other hand, the emphasis on the importance of feeling also reflects a distinctive view of the cognitive realm that stresses the role of spontaneous value attribution.

In the Abhidharma, a mental state is not just an awareness of an object but is at the same time an evaluation of the object. This evaluation is the function of the feeling tone that accompanies the awareness and experiences the object as either pleasant, unpleasant, or neutral. This factor plays a central role in determining our reactions to the events we encounter, since for the most part we do not perceive an object and then feel good or bad about it out of considerate judgments. Rather, evaluation is already built into our experiences. We may use reflections to come to more objective judgments, but reflections mostly operate as correctives to our spontaneous evaluations. In the Abhidharma, spontaneous evaluation is based on the way in which the object feels to us. This is the function of feeling; the Abhidharma compares it to the king who tastes the food prepared by his retinue (the other mental factors).[23] This factor is also depicted as having a very close connection to some of the afflictive (and affective) factors we will examine shortly.

Feeling is not, however, the only important factor, and several others deserve a brief mention. Intention *(cetanā, sems pa)*, for instance, is a central and omnipresent factor that determines the moral (not ethical) character of the mental state. Every mental state approaches its object with an intention, a motivation that may be evident to the person or not. This intention determines the karmic nature of the mental state, whether it is virtuous, nonvirtuous, or neutral. Intention is associated with the accomplishment of a goal and hence is also thought of as a focus of organization of the other factors. It is compared with the head carpenter who makes the other carpenters work while doing his own task.

Also significant are three factors particularly relevant to the discussion of meditative states. The first one is attention *(manasikāra, yid la byed pa)*, one of the five omnipresent factors. It is the ability of the mind to be directed to an object. Bikkhu Bodhi explains: "Attention is the mental factor responsible for the mind's advertence to the object, by virtue of which the object is made present to consciousness. Its characteristic is the conducting of the associated mental states to the object. Its function is to yoke the associated mental states to the object."[24] Every mental state has at least a minimal amount of focus on its object. Hence, attention is an omnipresent factor.

This is not the case for two other related factors, concentration *(samādhi, ting nge 'dzin)*, the ability of the mind to dwell on its object single-pointedly, and mindfulness *(smṛti, dran pa)*, also translated as recollection, which is the mind's ability to keep the object in focus without forgetting, being distracted, wobbling, or floating away from the object. These abilities are not present in every mental state. Concentration differs from attention in that it involves the ability of the mind not just to attend to an object but to sustain this attention over a duration. Similarly, mindfulness is more than the simple attending to the object. It involves the capacity of the mind to hold the object in its focus, preventing it from slipping away in forgetfulness. Both factors, which are vital to the practice of Buddhist meditation, are included among the determining factors. They are not omnipresent but are present only when the object is apprehended with some degree of clarity and sustained focus.

The discussion of mental factors cannot, however, stop here, for we have yet to see how the Abhidharma conceptualizes the states we would describe as emotions. To do this, we need to examine the ethically determined factors, starting with the eleven virtuous ones.

> eleven virtuous factors: confidence/faith, self-regarding shame, other-regarding shame, joyful effort, pliability, conscientiousness, detachment, nonhatred (loving-kindness), wisdom, equanimity, and nonharmfulness (compassion).[25]

Although there is a great deal to say about these factors, I will limit myself to noting the presence of several positive factors that we would describe as emotions, including loving-kindness and compassion. Both of these belong to what we would describe as the affective domain, though here they are understood not in terms of their affectivity but in relation to their ethical character.[26] Thus they are grouped with other factors, such as wisdom and conscientiousness, that are more cognitive than affective. In the Abhidharma, all of these factors are grouped together. They are all positive in that they promote well-being and freedom from the inner compulsions that lead to suffering.

This is precisely the nature of the last group, the afflictive factors. This group is by far the most numerous, clearly a major focus of the typology. This group is also where we find most of the states we would describe as emotions. Here is the list:

> six root afflictions: attachment, anger, ignorance, pride, negative doubt, and mistaken view
> twenty branch afflictions: belligerence, vengefulness, concealment, spite, jealousy, avarice, pretense, dissimulation, self-satisfaction, cruelty, self-regarding shamelessness, other-regarding shamelessness, mental dullness, excitement, lack of confidence/faith, laziness, lack of conscientiousness, forgetfulness, stinginess, incorrect perception.[27]

Here again we notice that the list contains factors that seem quite different from each other. Some factors, such as ignorance, are clearly cognitive, whereas others, such as anger and jealousy, are more affective. The Abhidharma groups them all together, however, because they are all afflictive. They trouble the mind, making it restless and agitated. They also compel and bind the mind, preventing us from developing more positive attitudes. This may be obvious in the cases of attachment and anger, which directly lead us to dissatisfaction, frustration, and restlessness. Ignorance—that is, our innate and mistaken sense of self—is less obviously afflictive, but its role is nevertheless central in that it brings about the other more obviously afflictive factors.

Before moving on, I want to reflect on my first point, the nonexistence of emotions in the Abhidharma. As we have seen, there are many elements in the typology that we can identify as emotions: anger, pride, jealousy, loving-kindness, and compassion. But no category relates directly to our notion of emotion. Most of the positive factors are not what we would call emotions, and though most of the negative factors are affective, not all are. For example, ignorance and negative doubt are not emotions. Similarly, desire or attachment is not usually understood as an emotion, though this would be worthy of further discussion. Hence it is clear that the Abhidharma does not recognize the concept of emotion. There is no Abhidharma category that can be used to translate our concept of emotion, and our concept of emotion is difficult to use in translating the Abhidharmic terminology. The Abhidharmic way of cutting the pie of the mind is different from the Western typologies in which the concept of emotion appears. It emphasizes the distinction between virtuous and afflictive factors rather than opposing rational and irrational elements of the psyche.

Emotions and Their Remedies

The Abhidharma is not content just to make these distinctions. It also explains the genesis of these factors and offers a rich array of remedies. In examining the genesis of afflictions, the Abhidharma focuses on the close connection between the afflictive factors and feeling. The omnipresent factor of feeling is at the root of our spontaneous evaluative attitudes and has a close connection to what we would describe as emotions. In the Abhidharma, this connection between feeling and spontaneous evaluations is the starting point of the pathological reactions that lead us into suffering. For when we have a pleasant experience, we do not consider it as a fleeting expression of our sentiency. Rather, on the basis of our innate sense of self, we appropriate the feeling and get attached to it, wanting to extend it and intensify its pleasantness, while fearing separation from it. Similarly, we react with anger and aversion when we encounter an unpleasant feeling. We see this unpleasant experience not just as something we don't like but as a threat to our "self," and we seek to protect ourselves from it by rejecting it as strongly as possible. In this way, we get upset and entangled in our strong reactions of rejection.

Let me emphasize that according to the Abhidharma the problem is not the pleasant or unpleasant feelings, for they are just part of our being sentient. They are necessary to life, since without them we could not make the evaluations necessary to our survival. We do not function in the world as a computer, considering all the options and choosing the right one. Rather, we act mostly on the basis of our spontaneous reactions to experiences, and there is nothing wrong about this. There is also nothing wrong about our taking action to address the problems we experience. But actions require motivating factors, which are often affective in nature, and this is the crux of the problem. Although it is not the case that all spontaneous affective reactions are negative, some clearly are. Hence, it is crucial that we distinguish positive from negative states, as the Abhidharma does. But it is also crucial that we become aware of the ways in which these spontaneous negative reactions occur. It is here that the crucial link with feeling intervenes.

As sentient beings, we have pleasant and unpleasant experiences on the basis of which we act. The problem comes from the fact that we tend to overreact, getting attached to pleasant feelings and violently rejecting unpleasant ones. These attitudes are not necessary to our evaluative capacities but are pathological overreactions. I do not need to be obsessed about Italian espresso to be able to obtain it. I just need to notice the extremely pleasant feeling coming out of this delicious brew and take appropriate action. Similarly, I do not need to rant and rave about my political nemesis. I just need to understand the harm that he is bringing about and take action accordingly. Instead, however, I react with attachment or anger, in the process exaggerating the pleasing or unpleasing aspect of the object of my experience and constructing a web of emotional and cognitive entanglements. My coffee is not just good and my political nemesis not just a bad leader; they come to acquire for me extraordinary proportions and to occupy my thoughts. Moreover, these attitudes do not arise because I choose to entertain them out of considerate judgments. They just come on their own and take over my mind. Being deeply engrained in me, they arise automatically, without my having much choice, even when I know better. This is why we called them afflictive factors.

In the Abhidharma this connection between feelings and afflictions is crucial. It is here that, on the basis of our misapprehension of the self, we become entangled in the compulsive attitudes that lead us into suffering. But since these attitudes are not in our control, just wishing them away will not do. To be free from these pathologies, we must find ways to transform our cognitive process. This is where the Abhidharma's analysis of the mental factors acquires its practical significance. It is not just theoretical but informs and supports the numerous types of meditation recommended by the Buddhist tradition as remedies to the pathologies mentioned above. When one puts these remedies into practice through meditation, the obstacles to well-being, the afflictive factors, are removed and the virtues that constitute the good life are developed.

The meditative practices operate in various ways, but they can be summarized under two rubrics. Some meditations are the antidotes to negative factors. They counteract the negative factors by developing an opposed positive attitude, following Spinoza's dictum that "a sentiment cannot be restrained nor removed except by an opposed and stronger sentiment."[28] For example, the meditation on loving-kindness is described as opposing anger. Similarly, the meditation on impermanence opposes attachment. These antidotes have the effect of undermining the attitudes they oppose. When I suffuse my mind with a loving attitude, anger has no place; it is pushed back, suppressed for the time being. But although the results of this practice extend beyond the meditation, such meditations cannot provide a final solution to the anger problem. Anger may be undermined, but it will eventually return unless something more drastic is done.

It is this more radical approach that is at the heart of the second category of meditative practices, which are more specific to the Buddhist tradition. These practices do not just suppress the undesirable attitudes but eventually remove them entirely from our stream of consciousness. This liberation from the afflictions is in fact the goal of Buddhist practice. It is to be achieved by a threefold training in morality, the observance of precepts; concentration, the development of a focused and mindful attitude; and wisdom, the liberatory insight developed on the basis of concentration and mindfulness.

This liberatory process revolves around the strengthening of some of the factors we have examined. For example, the practice of single-pointed concentration strengthens our ability to focus on the object of our choice and thus strengthens the mental factor concentration, though other factors, such as attention, conscientiousness, and pliancy, are relevant as well. Such strengthening is particularly the case for mindfulness, the ability to keep an object in focus without forgetting the object or being distracted. Mindfulness is seen as being particularly important for dealing with the feeling afflictions, because by developing mindfulness we will be able to interrupt the connection to our afflictive feelings. And although this may not yet be the final goal, it is an important step in bringing about the kind of freedom that Buddhists seek in their practice.

The ultimate freedom is brought about by the sustained development of insight into the nonexistence of the self. When we become impregnated with this view, the very root of the afflictions, self-grasping, is weakened and eventually entirely eliminated. In a mind freed from the idea of self, there is no basis for attachment or aversion, there is nobody to be attached to and nobody to protect through anger. The attainment of such a state of mind is the fulfillment of the liberatory program of the Abhidharma; it is the state of ultimate mental health, where the pathologies of the afflictive factors are eliminated. Such a person is then free to entertain more positive attitudes, particularly the virtuous factors, such as loving-kindness and compassion.

Concluding Questions

My brief overview of a Buddhist view of mind and the way the Abhidharma tradition views the affective realm raises several questions, perhaps even challenges, which I offer as a conclusion.

First, it should be clear that the Abhidharma has a very different understanding of the mind in general and of the affective domain in particular. The Abhidharma does not recognize states such as anger, jealousy, or compassion as forming a category separate from the other functions of the mind. This does not mean that the Abhidharma ignores these factors; rather, it integrates them into other ethically determined categories. How does this phenomenology of the affective life compare with the ways in which modern scientific disciplines understand emotions? Is it really important to understand the affective domain as being made up of bursts of discrete and short-lived events, or would it be more helpful to think about a larger domain in which emotions are integrated into other cognitive functions, with possible ethical ramifications?

Second, what light can modern scientific disciplines, such as neuroscience, throw on some of the crucial points made by the Abhidharma, such as the connection between sensations and afflictions? These negative factors often can be quite destructive, and so developing ways to deal with them is important. Can these modern disciplines help illuminate ways in which humans can deal with this connection in order to gain greater freedom? And more generally, can these disciplines contribute to explaining further how some of the Buddhist practices can be effective in counteracting some of the af-

flictions? Finally, is there any possibility of finding neurological correlates to the distinction between virtuous and afflictive factors? Is this a
purely philosophical distinction, or does it have a neurological basis?

Third, as we have seen, the Abhidharma is based on a strong ethical distinction between positive and negative states. For me, this ethical emphasis raises a question: Is it possible to divorce the study of affects from ethical concerns? Affects are born from our evaluative
attitudes, spontaneous or not. Hence, they are laden with values. Is it
possible to study the affects born from these evaluations without considering the values that they reflect? And if we do have to consider values in the study of emotions, can we then ignore ethical considerations?

RICHARD J. DAVIDSON

Emotions from the Perspective of Western Biobehavioral Science

In the following pages I would like to accomplish four things. The first is to describe some key conceptions of emotion provided by Western science. The second is to begin to respond to the radically different conceptualization of emotion offered by Georges Dreyfus and in the dialogue with the Buddhists. The third is to raise some fundamental questions posed by this juxtaposition of the Buddhist view and the Western scientific understanding of emotion. And fourth, I would like to describe some new findings that we have obtained in our experiments with Buddhist monks that may bear on some of those questions.

In terms of how emotion is generally viewed in the Western scientific tradition, there are three aspects I want to focus on. We think of it as a mental state with a *valenced quality*, which means that it may be positive or negative. We think of it as a state often associated with a *bodily reaction*. And we consider it to be generally associated with

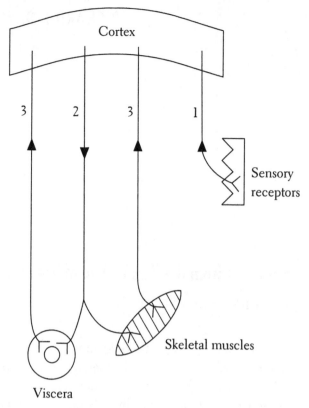

Figure 8.1 A graphic depiction of the James-Lange theory
of emotion, emphasizing feedback from the body to the
brain in the experience of emotion.

outward *expressive signs*.[1] For many of us, Western scientific ideas
about emotion take as their starting point the work of William James,
whose long chapter on emotion in his 1890 *Principles of Psychology*
has been very influential. There James presents a view of emotion
that emphasizes in particular the importance of the bodily response,
as illustrated in Figure 8.1.

The figure illustrates a process that begins with information coming into the brain (cortex) through sensory receptors (the eyes, for example). According to James's theory, the brain decodes the infor-

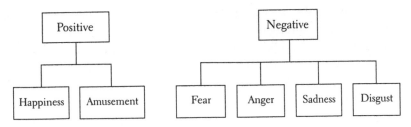

Figure 8.2 Valence model of emotion.

mation and sends appropriate signals down to the body: to visceral organs, like the heart, and also to the skeletal muscles in the arms and the legs. The body reacts, sending signals from the viscera and muscles back up to the brain, and it is the brain's interpretation of these bodily signals that constitutes emotion.

As James once said, we don't see a bear and then experience fear and then run. Instead, we see the bear, start running and feel our heart beating, and then feel fear, which arises from our conscious perception of the bodily changes. This view, which has come to dominate Western conceptions of emotion, underscores the central role of the body in our understanding of emotion.

A key question that Western scientists have asked is whether emotions are discrete and categorical, or whether they are more dimensional, smoothly blending one into the other. There are some emotions, like happiness, sadness, anger, fear, and disgust, that are considered by many psychologists to be basic and universal and also generally thought to be discrete and categorical. Paul Ekman has been a pioneer in the study of emotion from this perspective.[2] Discrete emotions like these are further said to be associated with equally discrete and distinctive facial and vocal markers. For this reason, some scientists have investigated how facial expressions can be used as signposts to signify the presence of a particular emotion.

At the same time, one can see each individual emotion as having a very small number of dimensions. The two dimensions that have been most emphasized are valence—the positive/negative distinction (see Figure 8.2)—and arousal, which refers to the strength of the emotion in question, ranging from very calm to very energized or active.[3] We are beginning now to consider the challenge posed by interactions with our Buddhist colleagues—namely, that Western science may have overlooked another important dimension of emotion: virtuous versus nonvirtuous or afflictive.

It would be a radical step for Western science to include this new dimension in its conventional model. To show just how radical, let me clarify more fully the traditional two-dimensional concept of emotion. It is a model organized around the two axes of valence and arousal (see Figure 8.3). At the top end of the arousal axis, emotions are very highly activated. Along the valence axis, high-arousal emotions may range from nervousness on the negative or unpleasant side to elation or delighted excitement on the positive (pleasant) side. At the bottom end of the arousal axis, we find "deactivated" emotions like calmness and serenity on the positive side, and depression and fatigue on the negative side. It is important to note that, to date, most research on emotions has focused on the valence and arousal dimensions of negative emotions, such as fear, anger, sadness, and disgust. Positive emotions have been much less well studied; indeed, only two have been studied with any seriousness: happiness and amusement.

How would our model look if it took on the challenge from Buddhism? A Buddhist-inspired model, reflecting an interest in how emotions parse along a virtuous versus nonvirtuous or afflictive dimension, would offer a very different way of mapping these phenomena. What would be the model's empirical benefits? Would our ability to interpret measurements of brain activity during different emotional states improve if we were to parse emotion in this new way? We do not yet have an answer to that question.

What about a benefit for those interested in studying the facial signs of emotions?[4] If we parsed emotions along the virtuous-afflictive dimension, would we begin to discover unique facial signs of virtuous emotions? Is there, for example, a facial sign of compassion?

In our laboratory at the University of Wisconsin in Madison, Matthieu Ricard, a Buddhist monk and one of the speakers at this

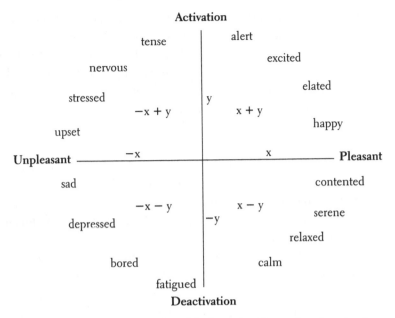

Figure 8.3 A two-dimensional model of emotion illustrating the role of valence and activation (or arousal).

conference, submitted to a series of studies that involved measuring his brain activity while he performed specific meditative practices. For example, in one study he was instructed to generate what Buddhists call "pure compassion," a very well practiced skill in the Tibetan Buddhist monastic tradition. On receiving the instruction to generate compassion, his face changed: the corners of his lips raised slightly and his eyes contracted slightly; both facial signs of positive emotion. This was itself interesting, because these facial signs do not map onto any of the already characterized facial signs for basic emotions; but our findings did not stop there. In the Western tradition it has been said that facial expressions of emotion never last for more than three or four seconds, but we observed something quite different in Matthieu's case. The distinctive facial signs in question persisted; indeed, they did not change throughout the entire period during which we were recording his brain activity. So already we begin to see the potential for our engagement with Buddhist practice to pose productive challenges to assumptions of Western biobehavioral science. It is important to note that these facial signs of compassion may not be universal, as other adepts do not consistently display them. What role they may play in generating the state of compassion is an issue that should be addressed in future research.

Matthieu and the other lamas who have participated in our research have helped us answer another important question as well: what impact does training the mind have on brain signals associated with emotion? The nature of the collaboration between our researchers and the lamas has been extremely unusual. Our visitors have become coexperimenters with us—not just subjects but collaborators in every sense of the word.

With their help, we began our research with a very simple design. We were interested, first, in comparing a neutral state with a meditation state, so we alternated a neutral state with a meditation state several times while the adept practitioners were either wired up for brain electrical monitoring or in the MRI scanner.[5] Even anecdotally, it was clear that this was not going to be business as usual, for after spending more than three hours in the MRI scanner, Matthieu came out smiling. Most people do not come out that way.

We then attempted to measure brain activity during a state of mind called "open presence." This is a term better defined by others with more knowledge, but we understood it to refer to a cultivated state of pure awareness during which the mind doesn't get pulled by emotions or by other external or internal events that are occurring. During the generation of open presence, we found a change in an area of the brain that normally assigns emotional value. Usually when a person receives a stimulus or has a thought, there is a reaction in which the stimulus is classified as positive or negative. During open-presence meditation, however, the part of the brain that normally assigns this kind of emotional value—the orbitofrontal cortex—was diminished in its activation. All six of the adept practitioners that we tested in our laboratory showed this change. For the first time, we have data from a whole group of adepts.

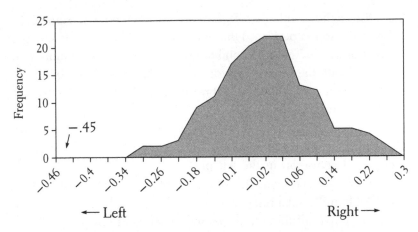

Figure 8.4 Histogram of the distribution of asymmetric prefrontal activation among a normal sample of individuals untrained in meditation. Measurement for trained meditator (far left) during the generation of a state of compassion is off the curve.

From here, we turned to brain measurements associated with practices supposed to generate compassion. Figure 8.4 offers a metric of brain activity from one of our subjects. The distribution curve in the figure, based on previous studies in our laboratory, shows the frequency of different points of activation for a group of 150 untrained subjects. Among these subjects, left-side activation in prefrontal regions at the points recorded on the chart was associated with increased levels of certain positive emotions. The data point for our trained subject is off the curve completely. Compared with the normal distribution pattern for untrained individuals, the pattern of brain activity in the adept practitioner generating compassion was so extreme that it was beyond that of any untrained person among the 150 that we had tested before.

We performed another experiment that was similar. With our trained subjects in either a neutral state or a meditation state, we presented certain stimuli designed to challenge their emotions. It was like a cardiac stress test for the emotional brain. While they were in meditation in the functional MRI (fMRI) scanner, we played for them the sound of either a baby laughing or somebody screaming, to see how the sound perturbed the mind. We found a series of changes in areas of the brain that respond to emotion. In the meditation state compared with the neutral control state, we saw a decrease in activation in those areas of the brain that normally react specifically to these emotion-arousing sounds.

We played the same sounds during the generation of compassion and found a similarly unusual reaction: the fMRI results showed an increase of activation in the left prefrontal cortex—associated with positive affect—in response to both the negative and the positive stimulus. We found similar responses with the brain electrical recordings. Taken together, all these findings pose a series of challenges to the usual assumptions in Western biobehavioral science.

Challenges are also likely to go in the other direction as well. Here is one that we in the Western scientific tradition would pose to our Buddhist colleagues: in the West, emotions, by and large, are conceptualized in an evolutionary framework. We know that even young toddlers and children display facial signs of anger and of fear. This raises some questions. What is the evolutionary role for what Buddhists would consider nonvirtuous emotions like anger and fear? Are these emotions perhaps important during early development, and then they become more destructive later in life? Are they always destructive, including in infancy and early childhood? Is there a way of seeing them as productive—virtuous—after all, under certain circumstances?

I'd like to push this last question further: several of my colleagues and I have been interested in the possibility that certain emotions, such as anger, that we normally consider destructive might contain some root component that is valuable; that can be used skillfully to overcome obstacles. Any emotion that is helpful to us in overcoming obstacles may be part of our evolutionary heritage, and it can potentially be distinguished from the evidently destructive and violent qualities that so often accompany anger in our culture. Is the destructive component of anger therefore a possible but not necessary feature of this emotion; something that has been learned through participation in our culture? In other cultures, is there an emotion that helps people to overcome obstacles but is not anger in the sense that we normally think of it—a skillful wrath, perhaps?

We are also interested in pursuing a cross-cultural dialogue about the role of consciousness in emotion. Some Western scientists make a distinction between feeling and emotion.[6] Feeling is when an emotion becomes conscious, but emotion may be the bodily reaction or the facial cues, which are not necessarily always conscious. In making this distinction, we then are moved to ask: what is the utility of an emotion's becoming conscious? Are we better able to regulate or control emotion when we become conscious of it? Which components of emotion are most available to our conscious experience? This question suggests that some components of emotions—the one most available to consciousness—may be more susceptible to modification through practice. Others, because they are more opaque and less available to consciousness, may be more impervious to investigation and to transformation through meditation.

Throughout this volume there has been a great deal of discussion about the complex role in the brain and behavioral sciences of first-person accounts of experience and of introspection more generally. One of the discoveries that Western scientists have made is that people who are untrained are very poor at giving accurate retrospective accounts of emotion. Untrained individuals are also not good at predicting how they will feel in response to some future situation. One important question for us is whether highly trained meditators are better at doing this. This is a question we can now begin to study.

There are other fruitful areas for interaction. Buddhists, we understand, make a distinction made between short-term emotions (that begin and end quickly) and more continuous emotions. Most emotion research has supposed emotions to be phenomena that are brief and episodic. But that may be changing. A growing number of scientists are beginning to suggest that emotions can be conceived of not just as states but also as traits.[7] By traits, we mean characteristics that endure over time. Traits often refer to temperamental qualities, like a person's being shy or very cheerful. These qualities persist over time and across different situations. This approach seems to be more consistent with

Buddhist thinking, and it and raises a further question: Can training change these traits? Can meditation be used to transform these traits? We're very interested in this because Western psychology often considers these traits to be relatively fixed and immutable.

The questions we're raising here suggest, in turn, a further cluster of questions. There is a concept in Western psychology known as "the hedonic treadmill." If a person receives some positive reward, he or she shows a change in his or her level of happiness, but the change doesn't last. It comes back down relatively quickly, and then the person wants more. In many ways, this is a Western model of craving and attachment. One example that has been studied is the experience of lottery winners. People who win the lottery and get a great big sum of money feel much happier for a very short period of time. Then their level of happiness begins to subside to where it was before. At that point they would need even more money to feel happier. The question is: Is there a way out? Is there such a thing as genuine happiness that is not subject to hedonic adaptation? Can happiness be conceptualized—and this is something very new for Western science—not as a state or trait, but as a skill that can potentially be learned?[8]

In his book written with Howard Cutler, *The Art of Happiness*, the Dalai Lama had this to say: "The systematic training of the mind, the cultivation of happiness, the genuine inner transformation by deliberately selecting and focusing on positive mental states and challenging negative mental states, is possible because of the very structure and function of the brain. But the wiring in our brains is not static, not irrevocably fixed. Our brains are also adaptable."[9]

We think he is probably right. At any rate, that is part of what we hope—through ongoing collaborations with our Buddhist colleagues—to find out.

Emotion

*The pair of presentations on emotion by Georges Dreyfus
and Richard Davidson provoked a slew of questions, both
from participants on the stage and from the audience.
Arthur Zajonc welcomed the two presenters into the
semicircle and introduced the panelists who would be
participating in the follow-up conversation: Daniel
Kahneman, professor of psychology and of public affairs
at Princeton University and recipient of the 2002 Nobel
Prize for economics; Dacher Keltner, professor of
psychology at the University of California, Berkeley;
and Daniel Gilbert, professor of psychology at Harvard
University. Matthieu Ricard would join with Georges
Dreyfus in responding to questions on behalf of the
"Buddhist side," Zajonc said, since Ricard and Davidson
were in the midst of collaborating on studies of emotional regulation.*

ARTHUR ZAJONC: I would like to thank both of our speakers for bringing us much closer to the theme of emotion as we see it from the Buddhist and Western perspectives. I would also like to underscore the significance of the long period of collaboration between Richard Davidson and Matthieu Ricard. We have just heard about a collaboration between a distinguished Western scientist in the study of emotions and a contemplative Buddhist practitioner who has also studied emotion and worked hard to bring those emotions into personal control. Thank you both for doing this extraordinary work together. You have already begun the collaboration we are envisioning.

We are going to turn now to the questions that have been raised. Quite a number of questions have been put forward, both by the Buddhist side and by the scientists. Georges Dreyfus posed questions to us concerning the phenomenology of the affective domain, and also concerning the neural correlates that might be associated with certain distinctions that are made in the Buddhist typology. He raised a large question concerning ethics, psychology, first-person perspective, and abstraction.

A number of questions came up concerning the role that consciousness might play in emotion. Why do we have destructive emotions at all? Is there some evolutionary reason for this? In the Buddhist context there is no comparable neo-Darwinian theory behind their understanding of emotion, but is there nonetheless a purpose to anger or other destructive emotions? There is also the question of traits versus states or skills.

We would like to begin with Your Holiness to see if you have remarks that you would like to make on these presentations.

DALAI LAMA: I had some questions but now I've forgotten them. *(laughter)* So let's start.

ARTHUR ZAJONC: Perhaps we can start with the question concerning the role of destructive emotions. That seemed to be an important one. I am wondering whether some of the other Buddhist scholars can speak to that. Matthieu, did you have something that you wanted to say?

MATTHIEU RICARD: About the notion of destructive emotions being necessary from the evolutionary point of view, you gave the example of anger. As you mentioned, anger might be useful for overcoming obstacles. In what way is anger totally undesirable, or at what point in the arising of anger does its negative, destructive, and afflictive effect occur? In general, if we consider our behavior, when hostile anger has developed in the mind, it is always afflictive, obscuring, and destructive. It disturbs our own peace and the peace of others. But if you look more precisely and carefully at the way emotion arises, all emotions, whether positive or afflictive, arise first from basic awareness, which is like a mirror that is not intrinsically tainted with negativity or obscuration. In addition, any emotion is like a musical note; it has several harmonics. Before it becomes afflictive, anger, for instance, has a quality of "clarity" or "brilliance." When we get angry, our senses are mobilized and our mind becomes sharp.

If we were able to simply recognize that clarity at the very moment it arose but not let it evolve in the chain reaction of multiplying thoughts that give rise to hostility, and especially to the strong distinction between self and others that creates the wish to harm, destroy, or reject, then it would not necessarily have a destructive aspect. Of course we are talking of very fine moments, and being able to remain in the luminous aspect of anger, without letting it evolve into an afflictive state of mind, requires great skill. Yet it is possible. Likewise with attachment, there is a moment before the blissful quality of desire turns to craving. This is very subtle; but the point is, from a Buddhist perspective, that the fundamental nature of mind is not intrinsically negative. Mental afflictions and toxins are not part of the basic, luminous aspect of mind. They are a deviation that arises when thoughts "chain" one after the other and become delusion.

ARTHUR ZAJONC: Is this aspect of the nonintrinsic nature of destructive emotions something that any of you would like to comment on? Do you see these afflictive emotions, for example, as having an intrinsic, biological basis that is somehow constitutive of what it means to be a human being?

DANIEL GILBERT: There's no doubt that emotions themselves have a biological basis. It's not clear that other animals have mental imagery or that they have control over cognition, but it is very clear that they have emotion. Emotion is generated by those areas of the brain that we share with all other mammals. And so I think the study of emotion is particularly important from the evolutionary point of view.

In Buddhism, certain emotions are labeled as disturbing or afflictive, and Buddhist practice helps us eliminate those. Fear is probably a good example. But evolutionary biologists have a word for animals that do not experience fear: dinner. *(laughter)* So emotions such as fear are very important.

The joke about dinner needs to be explained to His Holiness.

DALAI LAMA: My speculation, from the Buddhist point of view, is that to some extent the biological constitution of the different species might have an important role to play. Given the difference between the bodily constitutions of animals and human beings, we would expect to see different degrees of expression of some of these emotions. Similarly, even among human beings we see different traits, greater propensities toward anger or attachment among individuals. I would expect to see some biological basis for these. This is one way of looking at emotions, both destructive and positive.

However, there is another level to understanding these mental states, which from the Buddhist point of view we would expect to be much more universal, pervasive across all species, including human beings and animals. Buddhists would expect the presence of some basic emotions in all species.

Another point is the complexity of the issues involved when we are studying something like emotion, or even a single instance, like anger. It is very difficult to understand anger simply as a very short-lived, reactive, impulsive state that comes up from nowhere and then disappears. From the Buddhist perspective, mental states are understood as processes, which have a continuum, so that many other factors come into play. In some individuals anger might last long, but in others anger would be much more short-lived. For example, a practitioner highly trained in the cultivation of compassion may experience intense anger under a given circumstance, but one would not expect it to last long because of factors such as the strong practice of compassion.

So there are many factors that have to be taken into account. The biological constitution of an individual who may be more prone toward one emotion or another and environmental conditions all need to be taken into account. It's very difficult to understand the nature of an emotion like anger simply by looking at the state itself or the emotional expression.

GEORGES DREYFUS: I want to put forth a provocative little idea that is related to this. The problem with anger is not anger itself but the lack of freedom that we have. For example, if we entered freely into a brief burst of anger and then came out of it, that would not be a problem. In fact, I don't think it would qualify as anger. That is not what Buddhists mean by afflictive emotion, because the person remains in full control. The expression of a kind of wrathful energy would come out, but because it is under the control of the person, it would not be afflictive. It might help the person protect himself or herself, or accomplish what he or she wants to do. The deep-seated problem occurs when anger arises and we have no control. We are carried away. This is the real problem. The problem is not the emotions that evolution has brought about, but how we deal with them.

DACHER KELTNER: The Western scientific study of emotion has broken emotion down into many different pieces. We talk about the appraisal, the intention, the feeling or the sensation, and a tendency to act in a certain way and express it. The question I would turn back to you is: What is it freedom from? Is it freedom from feeling? Is it freedom from being obliged to act in a certain way? Is it a freedom from being aware of particular sensations? What does the training focus on?

GEORGES DREYFUS: The freedom is freedom from being compelled. The problem is not the sensation. The problem is not even the energy that arises in the person in reaction to the external event. The problem is how this sensation brings about a mental state that carries us away without any possibility of choice, and leads us to feel miserable and to be aggressive. The heart of Buddhist practice is the development of metacognitive skills that allow us to first notice this reaction and then channel the energy in a way that doesn't lead us to be carried away by these negative emotions.

ALAN WALLACE: There is a crucial issue here. In Western theology and philosophy, the existence of free will has been debated in tens of thousands of pages over a couple thousand years. Buddhists don't even ask whether the ordinary untrained mind has freedom of will, because it is so flagrantly obvious that we don't have complete freedom of the will. When somebody insults you, you may respond by expressing anger and resentment without any freedom whatsoever. It's obvious that we do not start out with perfect freedom of will. But the whole Buddhist path consists of cultivating such freedom, so that all your decisions are guided by wisdom rather than mental afflictions such as craving, hostility, and delusion. When you are enlightened, or as Ajahn Amaro said, when you are completely sane, then you are free to make wise choices at all times.

DALAI LAMA: I had not previously heard the point that Georges offered about the lack of freedom associated with destructive emotions. But generally we observe that one category of emotions is spontaneous, impulsive, and immediate. There may sometimes be circumstantial reasons, certain qualities of attractiveness or unattractiveness, that give rise to this type of emotion, but on the whole these impulsive, immediate emotions are very strong. At the same time, other types of emotions can be seen as reason-based, where as a result of a long process of contemplation, such as cultivating compassion, you arrive at a point of very strong feeling, such as the intense feeling of compassion. That kind of emotion is grounded in a more reasoned reflection. I feel that a distinction needs to be made between these two types of emotion.

RICHARD DAVIDSON: Would anger be considered spontaneous?

DALAI LAMA: Yes. In the first category of emotion, there is a lack of self-control. When these emotions come, they hit you; there is a lack of control and a lack of freedom. In the second category, regardless of how intense and strong the emotions might be, there is still a degree of freedom on the part of the subject. In fact, one can envision this type of strong compassion as a base that gives rise to a sense of disapproval and a strong feeling of something similar to anger, which could actually lead to a strong positive action. So here we can see the possibility of anger that is positive. This type of anger is different from the normal kind. Whether or not we call that emotion anger is a semantic issue.

DANIEL KAHNEMAN: I am impressed by the relationship between freedom and self-control. It seems that in this tradition, as in some others, including the Jewish tradition, freedom is self-control. You achieve self-control by freedom, and self-control seems to be a skill. Skill, we learn from research in psychology, is generally acquired through very long practice. A picture is emerging that you can probably train your emotions. But if it is like other skills, the psychologist Herbert Simon has claimed that acquiring real mastery of a skill may take up to ten thousand hours of practice. Of course there are many different kinds of skill, from chess to violin playing, and I assume a high level of compassion is a comparable skill.

DALAI LAMA: In some Buddhist texts there is the suggestion that it generally takes three innumerable eons to perfect compassion. *(laughter)*

ARTHUR ZAJONC: The question is whether the grant runs out before the end of the experiment!

DANIEL GILBERT: Like Danny, I was struck that the notions of freedom and self-control are very, very similar, and the benefits of that freedom are all too clear. They almost don't need discussion. I think an interesting question is: Are there costs? In psychology, the cost of the sort of freedom you are talking about is time. That freedom of the wisdom that one brings to acting or not acting on anger takes time—maybe only a moment, not ten thousand hours. But that is precisely why animals have emotions, because sometimes it's very important to act very quickly. If there is an unexpected movement in my visual field, I will feel a little fear and I'll move away. If you promised to liberate me from that feeling and bring it under my control, I would decline the invitation. I wonder if you could speak a little bit about whether in Buddhist philosophy there are any costs to the freedom that you are describing.

ALAN WALLACE: I would like to first add a correction. In the Buddhist understanding of the mind, if one had leisure to inspect the fifty-one mental factors with care, one would note something conspicuous for its absence. Fear is not among the six primary or the twenty secondary mental afflictions. Fear is not a mental affliction. Fear may be virtuous, ethically neutral, or nonvirtuous. In fact, there are certain meditative practices in which you cultivate a sense of fear that is based on reality in order to overcome that fear by taking the necessary steps to address it. The fact that we have so many Buddhist monks who survived to the present day suggests that they didn't become dinner.

The same is true of suffering. Suffering itself is not a mental affliction, even though that sounds rather strange. A mental affliction is defined in Buddhism as a mental process that disrupts, disturbs, roils, or warps the mind. If one attends to another person who is grieving and feels empathy with that person, that transient, empathetic sorrow is not a mental affliction. It is the fuel from which the flame of compassion arises.

Some suffering may be afflictive, some may be neutral, some may be actually wholesome. Likewise with joy. There is joy that is nonvirtuous or afflictive, joy that is neutral, joy that is virtuous. To return to fear, fear itself is not something that we are intent on demolishing right from the outset. There may come a point at which fear is no longer necessary, but that may take a while.

MATTHIEU RICARD: I wanted to say a few words about the notions of freedom and self-control. In the modern world we often think that the best freedom would be to do exactly what comes to one's mind. But in that case, we would simply be the slave of every single thought that arises in our mind. We would be just like grass on a mountain top that sways whichever way the wind blows. It would be like a sailor saying that freedom means letting his boat drift wherever the currents take her. We think of self-control as something that limits freedom, but in fact it's just the opposite: the true freedom of the sailor is taking the helm of his boat and sailing in the direction he wants to go, thus being the master of his destiny. Freedom from a meditator's point of view is to be the master of one's own mind and disentangle oneself from the chain reactions that usually keep on invading our minds. It's not as if we want to be free of the impulse to escape when we see a sudden threatening movement. That's fine; we are free to escape danger. But we are no longer free the instant that fear gives birth to a second and third thought of fear — when we are completely paralyzed by mental constructs of fear. At this point, fear becomes such a disturbing mental factor that we completely lose our inner peace. The anxiety born from this is not necessary at all and not useful: we have become the slave of the all-pervading fear that is imposing on our freedom.

The whole point of the training is to try to act on the moment when that chain reaction begins. There are many ways to do so. You can use antidotes. When the thought of anger arises, at that same moment you try to introduce a thought of patience, or compassion, or loving-kindness, because you can't have both the wish to harm and the wish to love at the same moment, toward the same object. They might alternate, but they are not compatible in the same instant. The more you think thoughts of loving-kindness and compassion, the less space your mind will have for anger and adversity. That's a very efficient and safe method.

Another method is to attack the chaining itself. When a thought arises, instead of powerlessly letting it multiply, just look at it and ask what is happening. Why should it multiply like that? In what way is it imposing on me? Is it like a weapon in someone's hand? Is it like a stone, or a fire in my chest? Look at it and experience the truth in front of you. When you look at it instead of letting it multiply, it just vanishes of its own accord, like the morning frost under the rising sun. The problem is simply that we are not mindful; we are not vigilant in the moment that a thought arises. We are not even aware of it. Of course it starts to multiply, and then it's too late. It's like a spark: it is very difficult to control a forest fire, but at the time of the spark, you can do something much more easily. So freedom lies precisely in not letting this fire of afflictive emotions spread throughout your mind. Freedom means that you don't let that chain reaction occur. As soon as a thought arises, it undoes itself, like a drawing made on the surface of water.

ARTHUR ZAJONC: One of the themes that has come up again and again concerns the question of trainability. Can we become more reliable in our retrospection, our looking back on emotional states? Can we become more conscious of our emotions overall? Can we transform our emotions? Can we become free? I don't know that we have a clear picture from the scientific side of how we understand what is trainable and what is not trainable. To the scientists, what seems to be intractable? How do you react to these claims concerning trainability and skill development?

DANIEL KAHNEMAN: It makes perfect sense from what we know about skill acquisition that this is a skill that could be acquired. If you repeatedly put yourself in situations mentally—clearly this is something that we can do—and you control your reactions time and time again, over a period of time, it may take many thousands of hours, but ultimately this is a kind of skill that could be acquired. There may be differences between the skill of controlling negative emotions and the skill of maintaining compassion. I was very curious about which of these you considered more difficult and more advanced. My guess would be that it might be easier to control negative emotions than to promote positive ones. This is something that I would very much like to hear about.

ALAN WALLACE: It really depends on the individual background that you bring to the practice. Some people are not particularly inclined to anger and lingering resentment. Others are very sharp, very easily aroused to anger, but it's very brief. When other people are aroused to anger it lasts a long time. Likewise for compassion. We see very young children who already display a natural propensity for compassion. For others it's much more difficult and takes a lot longer to cultivate.

RICHARD DAVIDSON: One of the challenges that we face in the West in this domain, as well as in the treatment of patients with mental disorders, is determining which individuals would benefit most from which particular practices, treatments, or training. Ideally, we would be able to learn something about a person that tells us whether a particular kind of training would be appropriate for that person before he or she actually begins it. Alan spoke about people who may have different propensities for anger; presumably there would be specific training methods for each.

MATTHIEU RICARD: Indeed, we say that we should first attend to whichever of the mental afflictions is stronger. That is the main task. Whether someone is more prone to anger or to craving, we should first concentrate on that particular afflictive emotion with antidotes and other means. That's why this is said to be a very flexible approach that depends on each and every individual nature and disposition. When we speak of 84,000 entries into the Buddhist path, it is precisely to emphasize the incredible variety of dispositions of sentient beings and the methods used to transform their minds.

RICHARD DAVIDSON: For those individuals who may not be particularly conscious of what their major style of affliction might be, is there a Buddhist manual of assessment?

ALAN WALLACE: There are many.

ARTHUR ZAZONC: Could you give an example of how a Buddhist abbot might assess the afflictions of one of his monks?

ALAN WALLACE: I was just reading a passage in one of the Buddhist sutras where the Buddha described how one evaluates another person by being with this person a long time, speaking with them, and examining their behavior carefully. It's not brain science, but it is behavioral science, using a very careful inspection to see what types of behavioral traits, characteristics, and tendencies people display. This is where the role of teacher, or mentor, and his relationship with the disciple, comes in. The mentor doesn't just give prepackaged techniques to everybody who walks in the door. Having carefully evaluated the particular predispositions of the student, the mentor hand-tailors the techniques for the individual. For example, in the attention training that I spoke about yesterday, there are not just one or two techniques. There is a wide range of techniques that are appropriate for individuals with particular proclivities or dominant mental afflictions. A person who is very strongly oriented toward anger and hatred will be encouraged from the outset to spend a lot of time cultivating loving-kindness, which is diametrically opposed to hatred and anger. Coming back to the issue of freedom, a person whose mind is compulsively prone to conceptual proliferation is encouraged to watch the breath as a way to calm the mind. Likewise for other typologies, there are specific techniques that have been found to be most effective for balancing the mind—not only the attention but emotions and cognition too—as a preparation for contemplatively investigating the nature of reality.

RICHARD DAVIDSON: The lengthy observation period that is required for this would certainly pose a real challenge to managed care. *(laughter and applause)*

MATTHIEU RICARD: There's an old story. There was a very famous nineteenth-century teacher named Patrul Rinpoche, who showed a way to examine a student's predominant afflictions. He came once to a hermitage where a hermit was meditating, and asked what he was meditating on. He answered, "I'm meditating on patience." Patrul Rinpoche walked around him and looked at him from all sides, and the hermit was a little bit nervous that this person had come to disturb his meditation. And after a while, Patrul Rinpoche said to the meditator, "Ah! Two frauds like us were meant to meet."

Obviously upset, the hermit said, "Why did you come and disturb me? I'm trying to meditate on patience."

"Hey, where is your meditation now?" Patrul Rinpoche said.

ARTHUR ZAJONC: I would like us to address one of the great ambitions of Buddhist meditation, which may speak to the core question of the hedonic treadmill. If one is looking not only for transient satisfaction or gratification but also for enduring happiness and a sense of true well-being, how can this ambition endure in the face of data showing that one again and again reverts to a lower level of satisfaction? It might be helpful first to say a little bit more about the Western understanding of the hedonic treadmill. Danny?

DANIEL KAHNEMAN: There are many results showing that changes in peoples' circumstances, including becoming richer or becoming poorer, or becoming married or becoming widowed, have transient effects on the happiness that people report. After a relatively short period, measured in months or in years, the level of happiness that people report experiencing returns to what it was. That is the main fact of the hedonic treadmill. But we also know that there are certain experiences that are not susceptible to the hedonic treadmill. Some pleasures of the mind remain and do not adapt. This is recognized in the Western world as well as the East. There are also some physical pleasures that we do not adapt to, that remain pleasurable forever. But the issue of the hedonic treadmill plays a very important role, because we seem to want things that turn out to do us no good in the long run. We engage in a great deal of activity to acquire goods that ultimately give us no happiness.

GEORGES DREYFUS: It's important to make a distinction when we talk about happiness, because this is a term that can be taken in different ways. Buddhism often says that the goal is happiness. But there's a very important distinction between pleasantness, joy, and well-being. It's clear that both pleasantness and joy are short-term, and probably most pleasant experiences are subject to the erosion that you describe. But the core meaning of the word *happiness*, in as much as it is promoted as a goal, is really a well-being that has the sense of freedom and of flourishing, and is not tied to any particular experience that is, by necessity, fleeting.

I would like to propose this distinction so that we can start to talk in a broader sense about what is implied by saying that the goal is happiness. Certainly the Buddhist tradition is keenly aware of the notion that pleasure is transitory. In my own experience, this was the first teaching I received from my first teacher, Geshe Rabten, who talked about this in the context of the three types of suffering. This understanding is very deeply embedded in the tradition.

ARTHUR ZAJONC: Before we turn to the audience's questions, are there any further comments from this side?

DANIEL GILBERT: So much of this meeting is about discrepancies between Buddhist and psychological conceptualizations. What Georges just said is a point of real agreement. It's very clear to psychologists that pleasures are transitory. What is interesting is that ordinary people have so little insight into the sources of their own well-being and happiness. Both traditions agree on that. There isn't a lot of mystery about why Westerners believe that transitory pleasures should last. We live in a consumer society. It's meant to maximize our consumption, not our happiness. We want to maximize our happiness and the society wants to maximize our consumption, and so we are taught that our consumption will bring us happiness. It turns out to be a lie, but we die soon enough and then a whole new generation gets to believe it. *(laughter and applause)*

DACHER KELTNER: The Buddhist practitioners have made an interesting point about the hedonic treadmill and why pleasure and happiness are so transitory that could really inform our science. We've thought about emotions as being very fast, object-specific reactions. You are talking about emotion as a state that arises through long contemplation. It would be interesting to hear about what those states are, what they are like in terms of their feeling. It's a window of opportunity for us to study.

ALAN WALLACE: In his presentation, Richard Davidson showed us a dimensional model of mental states in which alertness was correlated with high arousal and calm with deactivation, and similar contrasts were made between excitement and relaxation, elation and serenity. The Buddhist cultivation of attention leads to a state that seems to be an anomaly. On the one hand it is very alert, and yet on the other it is profoundly calm. It's not excited in the sense of being agitated, but it's very happy. At the same time it's profoundly relaxed and serene. You get both ends of the spectrum at the same time in an anomalous fashion, and that takes training. It's not the aroused attention of a video-game player, a fighter pilot, or an air-traffic controller. It's something different. This can be tested empirically.

DANIEL KAHNEMAN: In the literature on attention, there was an old distinction between two kinds of attention. The attention that is essentially oriented to action, or motor activity, is high-arousal; the attention that is receptive and oriented to accepting stimulation is low-arousal. That distinction is present in animals and in babies. It used to be a central topic in the study of attention some decades ago but has been lost since; clearly it would be worth reviving in the context of this conversation.

It was time to turn to questions submitted by the audience. Arthur Zajonc nodded to Anne Harrington, who would be reading aloud as many of these as possible for consideration by the group.

ANNE HARRINGTON: We have a lot of questions from the audience this session — I am holding nine questions in my hand here — and I have been struggling to organize and integrate them in such a way as to bring as many of them to the table as possible. My suggestion, therefore, is that rather than having a whole round robin of responses to each question, I will instead invite a response from the one or two individuals for whom a question might be particularly appropriate. Some of the questions seem to be aimed particularly at the scientists and some at the Buddhists, so we will go back and forth a bit. I'm going to start with the Buddhists, and I think that Georges Dreyfus might want to begin by taking a stab at this first question: "You say the mind is fluid, and that there is no king. But what do you call the meditator's 'I'—that which is doing the investigation?" We'll start with a hard one.

GEORGES DREYFUS: This is obviously a complex topic, but the goal of the Abhidharma is precisely to understand this process of meditative investigation in impersonal terms. What is doing the meditation is a number of factors that work synchronically or in interdependence with each other. The goal of the practice is to promote the factors that will lead to more well-being, to greater freedom, and so on. So it's not really "me," in any strong sense of the term, doing the meditation. We use this word, "I," because we speak conventionally, and there is no problem with that. And so, conventionally speaking, yes, "I" am doing the meditation. There is no denying that. But often what we mean by "I" has a much stronger connotation. So I would respond to the question, "What is the 'I' that meditates?" by saying that the "I," in the strong sense of the word, is what is to be eliminated by the meditation itself. *(laughter and applause)*

ANNE HARRINGTON: This next question opens up some larger questions about how ethics relates to methodology and the scientific enterprise more generally. I think I would suggest that Richard Davidson respond to it, at least to begin. Here is the question: "As Georges Dreyfus pointed out, in the Abhidharma the categories of virtuous and nonvirtuous are defined by ethical, religious purposes—that is, whether or not they lead to suffering. Can this categorization be used outside of this ethical context as a value-neutral categorization in the laboratory?"

RICHARD DAVIDSON: There are many ways to answer that question, but operationally we can certainly use the framework of virtuous and afflictive to distinguish between particular emotional states that might be generated in the laboratory. For individuals who are not Buddhists, or part of any particular religious or spiritual tradition, we can define virtuous, roughly speaking, as something that will lead to a reduction in those things that disturb the mind, that produce suffering, or that lead to agitation; and the opposite as afflictive. We can use that scheme to distinguish among emotions in a different dimensional framework than we have used previously.

ANNE HARRINGTON: But is it still a normative scheme, or is it a value-neutral scheme?

RICHARD DAVIDSON: I think it's difficult to use that scheme without implying some value.

ANNE HARRINGTON: This is a question that seems to be directed toward the monks who might be participating in future studies with scientists. The questioner notes that "scientific researchers would like to have a method of measuring constructs like compassion." She then asks: "But how do Buddhist practitioners know when they are in a compassionate state?" *(laughter)* In other words, are there any observable characteristics that can be measured? Now that we have brain-based, third-person indices that might reveal something about compassion, how can we start to measure and correlate those indices with phenomenological measures of compassion?

MATTHIEU RICARD: There are many kinds of compassion. Some are focused on a particular person or group who suffers and go together with empathy—that is, imagining vividly the feeling that the other is experiencing. Some are related to a state of benevolence that pervades the mind and is accompanied by a complete readiness to act for the benefit of others without necessarily trying to "feel" the suffering of others. In general, compassion is defined as the "wish that all sentient beings may be free from suffering and the causes of suffering." This goes quite far, since the causes of suffering include all mental toxins and basic ignorance. Likewise, loving-kindness means not just loving or liking somebody, but it is the wish that another person may find happiness and the cause for happiness. There are a lot of factors: the cause of happiness comes with wisdom. All-pervading benevolence excludes any thought that is self-centered, self-motivated, or limited to a certain number of beings. It is unconditional love and compassion. Once feeling loving-kindness and compassion, one may go on to examine whether such positive emotions are partial or all-embracing, whether they proceed from a mind free from delusion or are tainted with grasping. As to measuring its intensity, one may combine self-report with what is detected by the experimenters.

RICHARD DAVIDSON: In our work we actually do ask the monks after each meditation practice to scale their experience on certain specific dimensions that, in consultation, Matthieu suggested as relevant. I can tell you that there is variation across sessions. Not every meditation produces intense compassion each and every time. There is some variation represented in how they are scaled.

ARTHUR ZAJONC: Is the internal scale more or less in agreement with the external, measured result?

RICHARD DAVIDSON: That is a critically important question, and the honest answer is that we don't know yet. It's too early to tell.

ANNE HARRINGTON: This is a question for both Richie and Matthieu: "Was there any difference in Matthieu's response to the baby laughing versus the woman screaming?"

RICHARD DAVIDSON: The preliminary answer is yes, there does seem to be a difference. But it's very preliminary, and the data are still being processed. This is all very new.

ANNE HARRINGTON: You understand the implication, that a baby laughing would be something joyful and positive, and the woman screaming would elicit a different sort of response? Matthieu, what is your subjective memory of that?

MATTHIEU RICARD: Altruistic love and compassion are two facets, but they are not intrinsically different. We often associate loving-kindness and compassion as one basic feeling of all-embracing benevolence. When one is confronted with suffering, it arises as compassion. When one is confronted with the happiness of other, it appreciates that happiness and wishes that it may increase. It's like a complete readiness and availability to alleviate others' suffering and increase their happiness.

ANNE HARRINGTON: This next question is again for the Buddhists. The questioner asks: "What, if any, form of evidence coming from the Western scientists' work might you use to modify or incorporate into your training?" Or, to put the question a different way: Could you imagine biobehavioral data causing you to modify the way in which you practice? Or is the internal confirmation from first-person experience of the efficacy of the practice sufficient in itself?

MATTHIEU RICARD: In the course of the ongoing collaboration between meditators and scientists, we are trying to investigate more finely what happens during meditation. Any kind of feedback might thus help us to investigate the first-person view further and discriminate between mental factors or states that we have not been able to distinguish so far. Through further investigations, we might be able to make finer distinctions.

ALAN WALLACE: Even though the brain may not tell us much at this point about the effects of meditation, simply because it is so tremendously complex, psychologists have developed very sophisticated behavioral measures. Buddhists also make inferences about the mental states of students and so forth, based on behavior. There could be a great deal of complementarity in having another vantage point from which to evaluate whether a particular type of meditative practice is working. Having said that, there's also a cultural aspect at work here. There may be some meditative practices that have worked extremely well for twelve hundred years in Tibet. If you take exactly the same practices and try them in Boston in the year 2003, they may not work very well for quite a few people—not because the practices are no good but because the context is so radically different. Buddhism has gone through a process of assimilation and adaptation over 2,500 years as it has developed in different cultures. This is happening now as well. We want to make sure that these practices can be just as effective here as they were in Tibet and India in the past. This needs very careful research. Whatever help we can get is to everyone's advantage, not only for Buddhists but for all of us concerned with compassion and greater well-being.

DALAI LAMA: To follow up on Alan's point about cultural specificity, there are ancient non-Buddhist Indian traditions in which the notion of an enduring, eternal principle—an "I" or a soul or a self— is central to the spiritual tradition. Many of their contemplative practices for enhancing compassion or reducing destructive emotions are built around that philosophical premise. It would be interesting to see whether any neural or biological differences can be detected among practitioners who are cultivating the same emotion, like compassion or single-pointedness, but are grounded in a different set of philosophical persuasions.

ANNE HARRINGTON: I've got four more questions I am going to try to put on the table. Two of them are about the broader process of research, and two of them are about the implications of this work for nonscientists, for the general public. Here's the first of the first set, and I'm going to look in the first instance to the scientists for a response: "In using highly trained meditators as subjects, how should scientists account for the bias of self-selection? Highly trained meditators may have had well-balanced minds or special determinations to begin with. What do Buddhists think about the representativeness of these highly trained meditators?"

RICHARD DAVIDSON: It is an issue we have thought a lot about. A critic might say that some of the unusual findings we've obtained from the monks may have absolutely nothing to do with their training. If we were able to test them when they were young children, before they began the training, maybe they would show the same thing. That is a question we have not yet been able to answer. In response, we have been talking with Alan Wallace and Matthieu Ricard about doing longitudinal studies in which we would test people at different points during the course of training, so that each person could be compared with himself or herself before the training began. Only that kind of design will allow us to definitively eliminate the hypothesis that it's purely self-selection.

In work that Jon Kabat-Zinn and I have done, where Jon taught a simple mindfulness meditation practice to people who had not previously done meditation, we did test people before and after the two-month meditation program. We were able to detect changes in tests before and after that could not have been exclusively a function of self-selection.

ANNE HARRINGTON: We have been using the metaphor of Olympic athletes of mental ability. You can expect that every kid who is sent to gym class would become more fit, but you wouldn't expect every individual to have the ability to become an Olympic athlete. Maybe we will find a balance between innate ability and trainability. The fact that Steve Kosslyn has not yet been able to find an Olympic athlete of imagery doesn't mean that there isn't one out there.

Let me keep going with my questions: "What does the Western scientists' emphasis on not treating Buddhists just as guinea pigs but as collaborators say about our Western scientific treatment or attitude toward nonspecial subjects?" *(applause and laughter)* Any of you should feel free to jump in here. *(laughter)*

DANIEL GILBERT: It always seems like it's fun and funny to use the words *guinea pig* and laugh, as if scientists and psychologists treat people as mere subjects. But anybody who reads psychology knows that those who participate in experiments are treated with the utmost respect for their welfare and well-being, and that anything that happens to them in the laboratory is thought about carefully by the scientists and by a variety of governing institutional boards. So we may use the words guinea pig jokingly but perhaps we shouldn't, because it wouldn't be a joke if subjects were treated that way.

ANNE HARRINGTON: Here's a question that begins to open up the larger issue of the implications or usefulness of this sort of work for the general public. The questioner asks: "Have you done similar research on adept meditators who are not monks? It seems that if you could show these same results in lay people, we could benefit more people, because more people can relate to lay yogis or meditators than they can to monks."

RICHARD DAVIDSON: It's a very important question, and I appreciate the motivation of the questioner. We certainly would be extremely interested in this, and we have tested some individuals who are not monks. But in doing research of this kind, scientists prefer to study individuals who have all gone through very similar training. If we could find a pool of individuals who are not monks and who have gone through very similar training, that would be very helpful. We have been talking to Alan Wallace about studying longitudinal changes in lay people, not monks, as a consequence of going through a long-term retreat.

ALAN WALLACE: Like your project with Jon Kabat-Zinn, there was a project conceived at the Mind and Life conference in 2000 by Paul Ekman, which was carried out with Margaret Kemeny as the principal investigator. Margaret Cullin and I are the cotrainers for this project. We are teaching schoolteachers secularized versions of Buddhist meditations, but with little of the theoretical framework. Longitudinal studies are being done to see whether some of these basic practices of mindfulness, compassion, and loving-kindness, integrated with techniques from cognitive behavioral therapy, can help them in their daily lives, at home and at work. This research is ongoing, and the results so far have been very promising.

MATTHIEU RICARD: The criteria for inviting a person to participate in our studies was not at all whether they are monks or not. We looked at how many years they had been practicing. It just happened that many monks have been practicing for a long time. But we have also been investigating Western lay practitioners who have done many years of retreat. Whether or not a person is a monk is not an issue.

RICHARD DAVIDSON: We actually used the ten-thousand-hour requirement as an informal criterion. It limited our sample initially. (laughter)

ANNE HARRINGTON: This is a question directed now more explicitly to the Buddhists, and it also relates to the practical relevance of our work for people outside the academy. "You have argued that Buddhist mental training strives to bring about freedom. When more freedom is achieved through training, how does it translate into action? If there is freedom, there is choice. How does one choose with freedom without relying on valance or assigning different values to the option at hand? To go where one wants to go, doesn't it require wanting something, which is an attachment, or avoiding something?"

MATTHIEU RICARD: There is a difference between an aspiration and a desire. You may deeply aspire, in a selfless way, to do something beneficial for humanity; that is not a craving or an attachment. An attachment is something that limits your capacity to have wise judgments about how to bring well-being to humanity. This aspiration does not mean that you don't have any values or emotions. It's simply that those values and emotions are not afflictive. The basic values of removing suffering and bringing well-being are universal and fundamental. You can evaluate precisely how to use your freedom in terms of dispelling suffering and bringing happiness. I think that accepting those values would be totally acceptable and would not limit your freedom.

ALAN WALLACE: Georges Dreyfus has brought to our attention the triad of three primary mental afflictions: delusion, craving, and anger or hostility. His Holiness has already addressed the possibility of compassion inspired by anger that is not afflictive. Psychologists are well aware that some attachments are not afflictive, for example the bonding between mother and child, which is crucial for the child's survival and flourishing.

When Buddhists speak of attachment and hostility as mental afflictions, both of these have a common denominator: they arise from the root of delusion. In attachment, one is falsely, or delusionally, superimposing the source of one's happiness onto an object. In afflictive anger, one is delusionally superimposing the source of one's suffering on an object. Afflictive attachment and afflictive anger are both delusional, and in being deluded, one is not free. Freedom is essentially freedom from delusion, in which case one's aspirations and decisions are based on reality rather than on delusion.

DALAI LAMA: Similarly, although we reject the premise of an intrinsically real self, it seems that a positive sense of self is required in order to have strong self-confidence. An afflicted sense of self is much more constricting and delusional. Likewise, we speak of two types of desire: a positive, constructive one, which is nondeluded, as well as afflicted desire. The Buddhist tradition recognizes that at the beginner's stage, practitioners can even have spiritual states of mind, such as compassion, devotion, or faith, that are inspired by grasping at self or ego.

ANNE HARRINGTON: I just was handed another pile of questions, and as a result I have slipped two more from the new bunch into the short list of questions I'm still going to try to put on the table. I am holding in my hand now three questions that have to do with child development, and the age at which training of the sort we have been discussing might be introduced into someone's life. One of the questioners asks about the potential for introducing meditative techniques into the school system, and how early children can be introduced to such techniques. He or she is very practical. "How do we begin? How might we do this?" Another questioner is interested in how adults and parents in Buddhist cultures train their own children in these practices: "What age do meditative techniques begin? Do children trained in this tradition exhibit significant emotional differences from other children?" Our third questioner pushes the general theme further: "We are trying to be very practical in this dialogue. We want to use this information to change humanity toward a path of goodness. So in this sense, can the contemplatives on stage here comment on the techniques used by lay Buddhists in raising their children, in the home or in the school system? If the training were started in the home or at elementary-school age, we would all begin our adult lives with a greater baseline virtuous temperament." So we have here a set of questions that all have to do with the training of children, both in our own culture and in Buddhist cultures.

MATTHIEU RICARD: In Tibetan society it's not really done in a systematic way, but it comes naturally because children are exposed very early to a certain way of life and to people who are used to practice. Even lay families in Tibetan society engage every day in prayers and meditation, trying to transform their minds and become better human beings. It's something that children are exposed to very early, and it is quite remarkable how young children can learn something from that.

Of course, we are often surprised to see very young novices in the monasteries. It's not that their parents have dumped them there and they are crying and want to get out. Most of the time they are happy to go there, as if going to school but in a very serene atmosphere. I must say, I am quite struck when I pass by a school in Paris, at how much noise there is between the classes, with everybody running and fighting. We don't see that in the monastery. Among the seventy young novice monks who are in training in the monastery where I live in Nepal, it's extremely rare to see fighting or extreme outbursts of emotion. There must be something that is favored at a very early age by exposure to a more serene, peaceful, and loving environment.

I think the best approach is when the parents themselves are practitioners. The strength of example is bound to work the best, naturally, in every daily activity and in the way parents relate to and speak to their children. One of my own teachers, whose grandfather was also a very great teacher, told me that at the very beginning of his life he just saw his grandfather as a very kind and loving person. Slowly, as he grew older, he also began to discover the qualities of a great spiritual teacher in him. So it begins with teaching through human values, and then slowly cultivating and blending in the teachings and practice that lie behind those human values.

ALAN WALLACE: There is a remarkable school in Dharamsala that I have visited intermittently over the past thirty-three years, the Tibetan Childrens' Village. I have been struck every single time I have visited by the qualities of the two thousand children there, from orphaned babies in arms, to eighteen-year-olds who are about to graduate from high school. It's not a Buddhist monastery, but it's a school system where Buddhist principles are introduced very early on. The children are taught about empathy and compassion; there are monks coming and going intermittently who are role models. The children have their heroes, the greatest of whom, if I may say so candidly, is not a rock star, a basketball player, a muscle man, or a politician, but His Holiness the Dalai Lama. The people you admire are the ones you are most likely to become like.

GEORGES DREYFUS: I think the development of skills—emotional, cognitive, and metacognitive skills—is extremely important. In my own experience I didn't get all the skills I needed; my coming to the Tibetans, to His Holiness and all my teachers, was a way for me to acquire the skills I lacked. It would be really important if we could find ways that are not bound up with Buddhism or any other tradition to develop these skills. The obvious problem is the ten thousand hours. It ain't easy! But I think it's important for everybody.

MATTHIEU RICARD: At the same time, spiritual life is not like a vitamin supplement. You can play piano or not play piano; that's fine. We don't mind spending fifteen years to acquire knowledge and professional training; we go jogging for our health. But somehow we don't feel it's that important to spend time on inner development. That is very surprising.

DALAI LAMA: I would like to thank the three Buddhist speakers for their very glorified descriptions of Tibetan society but want to add that if you discount 10 percent of what they have said, it would probably be closer to the truth.

V

INTEGRATION AND FINAL REFLECTIONS

Integration and Implications

The final dialogue of the meeting was in some respects the most ambitious of the lot. While the first three dialogues had each focused on a specific topic, this last conversation was designed to be integrative: it was a time to look back, pull together loose threads, and address some of the large questions that had cut across the previous discussions.

This session also aimed to be an exercise in self-assessment. Had the fundamental premise of the meeting been borne out in substance, to the satisfaction of all concerned? Were we persuaded that we had here two approaches to investigating the mind that, working together, might achieve insights or be inspired to ask questions that neither, on its own, would achieve or ask? To help the group answer this question, we began the dialogue session by inviting MIT geneticist Eric Lander—who had been asked to listen critically to all of the preceding sessions — to offer us his candid assessment.

We believed that this final dialogue also offered the right moment for all of us to step back from our own immediate aspirations and put them in a larger context; to acknowledge the fact that this conference was not just academic business as usual. The conference had been "performed" (if one can use that term) on a stage before a packed house of some 1,200 people, and had excited much media interest. Most of this was connected to the involvement of the Dalai Lama, but what exactly did his participation in such a meeting really mean to all those involved? How should we factor any conclusions we might draw into our understanding of how to proceed with such dialogues in the future?

It was time to acknowledge other complexities as well: to talk about how Buddhists and scientists are not only similar but also different, particularly in the ways in which they think about what is possible and what is at stake in their respective efforts to investigate the mind. Differences in perspectives on the relationship between knowledge and ethics; differences in perspectives on the relationship between knowledge and the knower: all these ideas and more were fair game for discussion during this session. To open up these larger issues, following Eric Lander's remarks the conference organizers invited Harvard psychologist Jerome Kagan — who had also attended all of the weekend's proceedings — to voice his own reflections on behalf of the group.

First Lander took the podium and addressed the audience.

ERIC LANDER: I have no idea what I'm doing here. *(laughter)* I bring no experience whatsoever in Buddhism. I'm not a Buddhist, and I'm not intimately familiar with Buddhist teachings. I am also not a mind scientist — not a neurobiologist or a psychologist or a psychiatrist. I am, rather, a geneticist on the faculty at MIT, and my only qualification is that I am completely unqualified to make any technical comments of substance in both disciplines. For that reason the organizers asked me to serve more as a listener and member of the audience, to reflect on and integrate what I've heard.

Another reason why they asked me, as opposed to you (although there's still an opportunity for anyone who would like to to come up and do it!) is that I had the honor of spending a week in Dharamsala last October at the invitation of His Holiness, for another meeting on a different subject, the nature of life, which included molecular biology, physics, philosophy, and ethics. It was a truly remarkable experience, which they thought perhaps might help me to listen during this weekend. But I ask you to bear with me because it's a bit intimidating to summarize and integrate.

My first reflections are very easy. What an amazing two days these have been! I am sure that I speak for the audience in saying that it has been an extraordinary experience and a privilege to listen in on this remarkable and broad conversation. I want to say to all of the organizers, "Thank you."

Now I'll try to integrate what I have heard. I have organized it under five points.

The first: What are the foundations for any kind of dialogue between different traditions? The first foundation is a commitment to openness, to debate, to evidence, to a nondogmatic approach, and to respect. What does it really mean to be open? It means to be willing to change your mind and say you might be wrong.

I will tell you very briefly about a conversation that took place in Dharamsala in October, on a subject having nothing to do with the mind. We were having a discussion about embryonic stem cells, a very complicated subject in this country. It led us to the question, At what point might an embryonic stem cell, or an eight-cell embryo, be a human being? We debated back and forth, and the Buddhists offered that the Abhidharma mentions that, through the meeting of two regenerative substances, from the mother and the father, consciousness enters and the being then becomes sentient. From that, one might reason that the being becomes sentient immediately at fertilization and that there would therefore be very serious problems with working with such a cell. That was the Buddhists' opening position. As more scientific discussion went back and forth on this point, it emerged that if you took an embryo and separated the cells, you got two people, not one. And that if you implant an embryo, there is no guarantee that you will get even a single person; you might get none, because most embryos spontaneously abort. Maybe it wasn't so simple. Maybe, in fact, there was a different interpretation. Maybe there was no negative karma associated with experimentation at that point. It was a remarkable moment for me as a scientist, hearing the Buddhists and His Holiness discussing this. No firm decisions or commitments were made, but there was an openness to considering those things. I must say, it would be wonderful if we could have such open discussions in this country.

It's not enough for the Buddhists to be open to rethinking. Science also must be open to rethinking. At its best, science is about constantly being in doubt and maintaining a constant humility about how little we know. In practice, day to day, that humility does not always emerge. We sometimes take positions that can seem, and in fact are, very dogmatic: the brain can't change; it doesn't grow new neurons. Pressed, we acknowledge that may not be true, and we have to constantly remind ourselves as scientists that we might be wrong about all of these points, and that it is the evidence that decides. That is the first basis for any open dialogue: a willingness to change our minds, to be susceptible to evidence.

A second important basis for dialogue is to understand the motivation that we bring to it—not that we must have the same motivation, but that we should understand our motivations. Thereto, another brief story from my visit to Dharamsala: my colleague Steven Chu, a physicist who has now gone into biophysics, asked, "Is it okay to do animal experimentation?" His Holiness gave an answer that has stuck with me. He said, "It's not that simple. I can't say right or wrong. There's clearly bad karma associated with killing an animal in an experiment. But there are two other points:

What will be the outcome fifty years from now? Will it have a positive benefit in the world?" I could understand that in terms of the Western notion of cost-benefit analysis. But his next point was very interesting. He said, "The other consideration is what is in your heart as you do the experiment. What is your deep motivation, quite apart from any long-term consequences?"

I confess we don't talk about this much in the laboratory, and few institutional review boards pose the question: Explain what is in your heart in doing this experiment. We wouldn't even know how to deal with that question, and it clearly matters a great deal. So it's worth asking what our motivations are. Not just with respect to one's karma, if one believes in that framework, but what are the motivations that you bring to any investigation and any dialogue?

I think there are two clear motivations here. Both science and Buddhism bring a motivation to ameliorate suffering in the world. They attempt to do it in very different ways, whether they ameliorate suffering primarily through a mental process or primarily through a physical process, but there is some of both in each. In addition, there is another motivation that's quite different. Many scientists are motivated by pure curiosity. Many of the things they do in the lab are driven by a curiosity about the world. In listening to the Buddhist scholars, I think that they, too, share that curiosity. There is a deep and abiding motivation to ameliorate suffering in the world, but they also think in terms of a purely intellectual curiosity about the world. There is a meeting ground in both of those motivations. The experiments that must result from a collaboration will involve both benefit to the world and satisfaction of a curiosity for two traditions that have been thinking for a long time. That's a foundation for some dialogue.

Point two: What can Buddhist scholars bring to scientific investigation of the mind? There are several possibilities, and I see different advantages and disadvantages to each of them. One, they bring interesting experimental participants with highly trained skills. In particular, my colleague Matthieu Ricard has offered himself for these studies. He has worn that wonderful EEG headdress, and has come out of the MRI smiling after three hours, although Matthieu always comes out smiling. These studies are quite remarkable, and Professor Davidson's work really shows how much science can learn by studying a highly trained, skilled experimental participant. There's a difference between highly trained participants and college undergraduates paid at ten dollars an hour.

That is only one small slice of what Buddhist scholars can bring. They also bring traditional practices that have been worked out through experimentation and careful thought over some 2,500 years. How should we regard such traditional practices? One way is to regard them as something like folk wisdom, the way that pharmaceutical companies might regard a folk remedy: they're on to something, and now we will work out what the real basis of it is. I don't think that is the right way to regard it. I am persuaded that we have every reason to regard Buddhist practice as a refined technology that could play a critical role in science.

The Buddhist tradition is not a technology for detection, like an MRI machine, but a technology for modulation, which is very valuable in science. We at MIT right now are very excited about a new technology called RNAi (RNA interference) that can modulate genes and cells, because of the ways that it will let us probe how cells work. I think there is evidence not only that the brain is adaptable, that it might be possible to train attention and emotion, but also that there are specific protocols suggesting how we might do so. We should value highly technologies for doing things, because they are very hard to come by. They take a long time to work out and are very valuable.

The Western tradition has also apparently developed technologies recently for training the mind in new, powerful ways. I refer specifically to the discussions of video games, which seem to have effects on attention. At the same time, video games seem to give us only part of what we would ideally want from a mind-training technology. The video-game training seems to fail to develop relaxation, meta-awareness, mindfulness, and the ability to multitask calmly, which I, for one, would very much like to know how to do.

Another thing that Buddhist scholars might bring to investigation is specific explanations of brain mechanisms—how things really work in the underlying physical substrate of the brain. The Buddhist tradition has its theories and its explanations. We have heard descriptions of six types of awareness, fifty-one mental factors, genuine happiness, compassion, and joyful affect. I'm not sure that the specific descriptions of mechanisms will prove that fruitful, because I am not sure that introspection can point us to mechanisms per se. But I should note that I am equally suspicious of Western ideas about how the mind is organized that have emerged from introspection. We need other ways to study how the mind is organized. I'm not sure that either of the two traditions will be able to bring explanations because, I think, we are very far from understanding the mechanisms. The work of the next decades is to explore much more richly the phenomenology itself. Let's first get the phenomena described well. As a molecular biologist, I know that we cannot describe mechanisms unless we are close to them. A description of how cells divide, ten steps removed, doesn't help much.

That said, the well-developed Buddhist traditions do bring us something very important. They bring distinct perspectives that inspire ideas and questions. Sometimes in science we make too much of the technology or the data. One of the most important things in science is what questions you ask. People have often revolutionized scientific fields simply by raising new questions or posing a question differently. In this we have a tremendous amount to learn from dialogue between fields.

Buddhism proposes different ways to parse the world. Western science proposes different ways to parse mental abilities. Their taxonomies differ. They are probably both wrong at some level. Nonetheless, the fact that you have two approaches that don't map onto each other is very valuable.

Buddhism also brings specific constructs to investigate. I do not routinely think about the stability and vividness of images. Yet they talk an awful lot about that, and it must mean something. We have got to come to understand what that stability and vividness is about.

I also noticed that both sides have brought different metaphors, sometimes based on their cultures. We bring a metaphor from the Western side of the CEO, the executive in charge of the brain. I am told by my colleagues on the other side that the Buddhists use the metaphor of a very weak king, with continual palace coups going on all the time. These are different metaphors and they are rooted in culture. That does not make them right, but their difference is valuable. This is not exclusive to Buddhism. Marvin Minsky and others at MIT speak about the society of mind, a chaotic society that, if you live in the university world, feels very reasonable and comfortable compared with a corporation.

We bring different perspectives on what is fixed and what is changeable or trainable: the idea, for instance, that we should think about emotion not just as a state or an unchanging trait, but as a skill that can be trained. That assumption overturns some of our usual ways of thinking, and I think it will prove to be very important. It raises the question of how trainable the mind is. How much can the training be generalized? I hope the panel will talk about that.

In addition, as Alan Wallace said, the Buddhist perspective has brought different goals. In the Western perspective we focus on mental illness and try to get to normality. But Alan asked, Why stop there? What about the upper end of mental health, Olympic-status mental health? I think it is a very interesting question. Why are we satisfied just to say you are not mentally ill? Why is it not, like exercise, something that one could get better and better at? None of this conflicts with science. We just don't happen to say these things to ourselves that often. I think these different perspectives are of great value.

The third point: What are the most fruitful areas for collaboration? I challenge our scientists and our Buddhist scholars to think specifically. To deliver on the promise of this will require specific research agendas, which will require specific, testable hypotheses and experiments. I hope to hear more about them. I was excited to hear of Richard Davidson's experiments and the beautiful data there. We need lots more of it from many more people. An important theme of this research agenda is to better connect the first-person experience with third-person observables. The MRI is a powerful technique for doing that. It in some sense validates each perspective in the other's terms. The panel will talk about the differences in the status of first-person and third-person observations that figure in both traditions. But if we were able to say that compassion corresponds to a portion of the brain lighting up, it would have a powerful impact on the way we are able to do science, to design experiments, and to understand things.

I would even go further. I would like to see the assertions about enhanced faculties tested in very concrete ways. I am impressed by the assertions about attention. They seem quite reasonable from all the discussion, but they ought to be susceptible not just to MRI tests but to many psychological and psychophysical tests. I wonder if the Buddhists might do a better job of designing those psychological tests, to show what they are trained to do well. The psychologists have designed a bunch of tests from their context, but some of them seem a little stilted. It would be very interesting to ask the Buddhists to design a test that would distinguish trained practitioners from untrained practitioners. That research agenda would be incredibly important in taking this discussion to the next level.

Fourth: What can Buddhist scholars gain from such a collaboration? We have heard several answers. Using modern scientific methods, the Buddhist scholars may get new answers to old questions. His Holiness referred to an old debate about how physical objects are represented as mental objects. Is it a one-to-one mapping? Is it a many-to-one mapping? Is it a one-to-many mapping? That is what I took the question about cutting the egg to mean.

And the Buddhist answer, after 2,000 years, is that they don't know—and they would like to! That curiosity might produce contributions to these debates and questions. It has been proposed by some that the Buddhists might be able to further improve contemplative techniques, for example through feedback on how a student is doing. They have been improving their techniques over 2,000 years, but, as with all things, it is likely that knowing more about them may make them better.

There is the potential that science will "validate" claims, although that's always very risky, because one does not want to stake the validity of one's belief system on some other set of measurements. But there is something there.

In some ways, the deepest answer to what Buddhist scholars can gain comes back again and again to benefit for the world, benefit for others. I think this is quite remarkable. If I were to ask most of the Buddhist scholars what their primary reason is for participating in this dialogue, it would be that they think such a program will lead to benefit for others.

Fifth: What can the world gain? Several things. Specific knowledge about the mind and the brain. The questions are very challenging and we need all the help we can get. But there are some other things the world can gain. I will speak now as a scientist concerned about our society. We live in a world where science is a very powerful and effective paradigm, and yet we know it does not contain all the answers to all human needs. As with any one-dimensional diet, consuming only science leads to malnutrition. The fact that science does not contain the answer to all human needs has produced in many people, in our country at least, what some have called a flight from reason: a rejection of science in favor of the appeal of fantastical things. Forgive me if I offend, but I am referring to pyramids and crystals and such things. This debate is remarkably different. It is not about any flight from reason, or flight from science. It is possible for science and Buddhism to recognize happily that science is only one way of understanding the world. It can be incorporated; it can be worked with; it need not be rejected. I think that is really important. Our world would be much better with debates that are based on respect and an attempt to understand. Science very much needs to be willing to participate in those debates, because it has much, but not everything, to offer the world.

What might society gain in the long run? We may actually help to alleviate human suffering. The U.S. surgeon general advises at least sixty minutes of physical exercise five times a week. It's not inconceivable that, ten or twenty years from now, the U.S. surgeon general might recommend sixty minutes of mental exercise five or six times a week.

In closing, it has been extraordinary to watch two great traditions in our world, fashioned over centuries in the case of science and millennia in the case of the Buddhist tradition, come together through people of goodwill and good heart in this open dialogue. For me, as I suspect for so many of you here, it has been a privilege to listen, and we are all enriched by it.

By mutual agreement, there was no discussion or question taking immediately following Lander's remarks. We wished to give both speakers the opportunity to say their piece before opening the conversation up to everyone. At this point Jerome Kagan rose from his seat in the semicircle and took Lander's place at the podium.

JEROME KAGAN: Your Holiness, ladies and gentlemen, the organizers were wise to pair us in this way, because my comments follow in a coherent manner Eric's wonderful presentation. I, too, applaud the wisdom and the courage not only of His Holiness but also of the Mind and Life Institute for arranging this extraordinary meeting and its rich dialogue.

I want to address two distinct questions. The first is why this meeting was oversubscribed so quickly. I'm suggesting that this would not have occurred fifty years ago, when Americans were confident and smug, when the good had defeated the bad and everything was clear. An answer to the "why now" question requires some historical analysis. The second, more pointed question is, can trained Buddhist introspection add substantially to our understanding of the human psyche?

I deal first with the suggestion that the popularity of this meeting is a result of the social changes that occurred over the past century, and those changes have affected our assumptions about human nature. The new descriptions of humans that emerged in Europe when the medieval era blended into the Renaissance were due to profound changes in political and economic structures. The changes that occurred half a millennium later, during the Enlightenment, were consequences of scientific and mathematical advances and Luther's bold challenge to the authority of the Vatican.

I suggest that, from the Enlightenment to World War I, most members of Western society did not question the ultimate truth of the following three propositions. One: Humans possess a free will that permits each individual to decide what to believe and what acts to implement or suppress. Therefore each person must assume responsibility when he or she violates a moral standard. I remind you that free will was a popular nineteenth-century idea and one could find this term in every nineteenth-century textbook. As Professor Dreyfus noted this morning, the notion of a mind able to control its emotions is also central to Buddhist philosophy.

Two: Although our basic sensory motor abilities and our physiology are inherited, making it difficult to change the content of our thoughts, our cultural institutions are created constructions that lie far beyond the reach of our genome and could not be predicted from human biology.

Three: Although humans inherit a biological bias that permits them to feel anger, jealousy, selfishness, and envy, and to be capable of being rude, aggressive, or violent, they inherit an even stronger biological bias for kindness, compassion, cooperation, love, and nurture—especially toward those in need—because this ethical imperative is a biological feature of our species. This is also the Buddhist premise. I can assure you, as a student of children for forty years, that developmental psychology affirms the validity of this claim.

A thought experiment is persuasive. I want each of you to estimate the total number of opportunities for all individuals across the world to commit today an asocial act—aggression, murder, rape, rudeness, dishonesty, robbery—with complete certainty that they will never be discovered or punished. Put that very large number in the denominator, and in the numerator place the number of asocial acts that will actually occur today. That ratio is close to zero every day of the year. If you place in the numerator the number of benevolent acts, leaving in the denominator the number of the malevolent ones, that ratio is greater than one every day.

Thus the human chimera is more lamb than lion, even though there have been brief intervals when philosophers, especially Europeans, were uncertain about that truth. Thomas Hobbes, for example, was far more pessimistic. But the Buddhist premise that we are more strongly biased to be benevolent rather than malevolent is probably a basic feature of our species. Most of you are here to find support for that belief because we have lived through a period of history that threatened that idea. This threat arose because history's Muse woke from her slumbers and, bored with the status quo, decided to stir the pot and see what new scenarios she might create.

First, she arranged new migrations in the middle of the last century that further diversified America and Europe at a time when the economy had changed and the labor of new migrants was not as necessary as it had been a half century earlier, during the late nineteenth century. As a result, vocational and class mobility were stalled and too many youths from immigrant families could not ascend easily to middle-class status. In reaction to that frustration, the Muse arranged for a raising of consciousness and guilt over previous prejudices toward these new citizens.

Those changes in consciousness required the privileged majority to acknowledge the dignity and validity of the values of all minorities, and, as a result, many began to question the truth of their moral imperatives and became uncertain about the meanings of sin and sacrament. The problem is that humans find it difficult to cope with this type of ambiguity. Once any one of us begins to lose our unquestioned faith in the moral veracity of the beliefs we acquired during childhood, we become unsure of the goals to which we should commit our passion. That mood of uncertainty is especially toxic to youth.

Moreover, the new moral imperatives for understanding and tolerance, and allowing the less fortunate to enhance their sense of virtue, required this society to select a goal that all might attain with effort, one that did not impugn the disadvantaged minority. Unfortunately, gaining wealth and status fit that requirement, for neither is a personal feature like ethnicity, skin color, national origin, or gender, which nineteenth-century Americans used to reassure themselves of their virtue. The choice of wealth and status as goals transformed many, especially in American society, from socialized, moderately tame pit bulls into solitary, stalking jackals. Humans do not like to think of themselves as jackals.

Dramatic advances in molecular biology, genetics, and neuroscience during the latter half of the twentieth century were the Muse's final intervention. A small but especially vocal group of biological scientists declared that the public had exaggerated the power of human will and the infinite possibilities of culture as sources of human benevolence. We had to acknowledge the powerful, but unfelt, biases that were inherent in our biology.

These historical events led many to question the reality of both sin and free will, and the traditional rationale for restraining self-interest and an aggrandizing ego. Many who reflected on the implications of this new form of Calvinistic predestination felt threatened. The public was being told that, while people had the illusion they were free to decide when and where to nurture or to attack, in truth the anatomy and chemistry of their brains, partly given by genes, were the true executive directors of their daily actions. Given this state of affairs, none of us should be surprised that many Americans became eager for any scientific evidence or philosophical argument that could challenge this dark, materialistic view of human nature.

Buddhist philosophy is one stance that a bold David might take in a battle with the twin-headed Goliath of biological determinism and the uncomfortable tension that accompanies the daily need to be competitive, self-interested, and suspicious of the intentions of others, rather than concerned with one's community and neighbors. It is as if we recognized the correctness of John Donne's famous lines: "Never send to know for whom the bell tolls; it tolls for thee."

The welcomed Buddhist view claims that joy and serenity are not slavishly tied to our physiology, because humans are not objects manipulated by biological forces but active participants in control of the generation of our thoughts and emotions. The Buddhists say you must treat the human mind as a coherent whole, rather than as a set of separate modular parts — a crimson sunset, not a collection of dust particles reflecting the dying sun's photons.

In contrast to the dictates of current scientific presumptions, the Buddhists insist that one cannot understand the human mind by analyzing it into its separate components without any value constraints. Humans are unlike any other animal. Reflecting on their past and its relation to the present, they are influenced not only by sensations but also by their notions of right and wrong and of an ideal. Humans are first and foremost ethical animals. That is a scientific statement, not a philosophical one. We are ethical animals who, unlike any other species, automatically evaluate our experience as good or bad, right or wrong.

Remember how you applauded yesterday when a Buddhist scholar said that an ethical stance penetrates every meditation. Most scientists, though not all, do not know how to deal with that claim. Nature, they say, is value-free: just the facts; no value judgments. When hyenas kill lovely gazelles, or when Hutu murder innocent Tutsi, we should understand—they say—that this behavior is consonant with the Darwinian principle of maximizing the fitness of each individual.

I suggest that the Buddhist premises are appealing because they are effective weapons against those who wish to reduce human psychology to neurons, transmitters, and protein receptors programmed to push all of us to look out for self first. I have some neuroscientist friends, whom I respect and play tennis with, who assume that the statement "Mary felt afraid when she saw the spider on her bed" will one day be replaced with "There was increased synchrony of neural firing at four to eight cycles per second in the lateral amygdala and hippocampus after Mary's thalamus and visual cortex registered the small black form on the white surface." That sentence was not meant to make you laugh.

An important reason for the popularity of this meeting is that most of you were feeling that historical events over which you had no control had deformed your basic urges, and you were eager for philosophical support for what your intuition told you was true.

My second question addresses the distinction between the philosophical assumptions of Buddhism and the methods of trained introspection. The primary purposes of this meeting were to consider whether individuals trained in the Buddhist form of introspection could discover significant new data about the human mind that no other method could reveal and, second, whether those data offered special or privileged access to more fundamental truths about reality. This separation is important because Buddhist philosophy has an ethical foundation. But true facts about nature are often inconsistent with ethical premises, a profound insight that Wittgenstein understood.

In this final comment I focus on the empirical facts about mind that introspection can uncover. I am not talking about the therapeutic value of introspection for the person seeking a more serene, compassionate state. Those states are different functions of meditation and introspection.

Although the Buddhists contend that specially trained introspection can reveal deep truths about the human mind that EEG or fMRI scanner could never discover, I remind you that Niels Bohr, the Danish physicist who is one of my heroes, suggested that no method has a uniquely privileged power to reveal the true nature of anything. It does not matter whether we record neuronal activity, behavior, latencies in a priming experiment, or the products of trained introspection. Each method reveals something different about the whole, and we need a variety of procedures to come closer to answers that, of course, we will never fully possess.

There are two reasons for this pessimistic claim. First, there is a wealth of robust scientific evidence demonstrating that some biological events, in principle, are not accessible to awareness—not even trained awareness—and those events influence our feelings and actions. For example, if adults are told to listen carefully to a series of sounds—*ba, ba, ba, ba*—and to report when they perceive any subtle change, they fail to detect consciously a slight physical variant of that sound. But their brain detects it, even if they're sleeping, and produces a very clear wave form in their EEG. Similarly, every time any one of us sees a friend, spouse, or colleague for the first time in the morning, a brief autonomic reaction occurs that is completely unavailable to awareness.

More important, the results of every method have a special form and are described with a distinct metric. The metric that communicates the products of trained introspection to others consists of categories, usually—but not always—semantic. These language forms are simply not fine enough to capture bodily events that occur in milliseconds in parts of the brain that are permanently hidden from the light of introspection.

Trained introspection is a lens with a fixed curvature. The lens can be polished and cleaned to make the perception more accurate, but unfortunately its focal length is fixed. A serious problem for trained introspectionists is that in order to communicate their insights to others, they must use words. Sadly, words were not invented to describe these private perceptions and sensations. Words were invented by *Homo sapiens* to describe categories of things in the world—animals, food, objects, people and their movements—or to instruct people as to how to behave. Most of the things that are described by words, neuroscientists tell us, are mediated by a special circuit. Words represent large, relatively coarse events that either stay still or move at a slow pace. Words are the worst possible vehicle to communicate private sensations that are mediated by a different circuit. Evolution separated the neuronal bases for these two sources of information. The task of describing most private experiences can be likened to reaching down into a deep well to pick up small, fragile crystal figures while wearing thick, leather mittens.

Even if the trained introspectionist were able to pierce the veil that hides the fast-moving, subtle changes that occur in brain and body, the person would have great difficulty in sharing that information with others. Perhaps nature wanted these feelings to remain secret, locked in each agent's sense of his being. I want each of you to reflect for a moment on the gap between the taste sensations that accompany eating French chocolate at the end of the day when you're hungry, and your linguistic account of that experience. Even Marcel Proust would have had a hard time. Recall Professor Wallace saying yesterday, "Well, there's a special state. You are aware that you are aware." To describe that feeling in words is almost impossible.

The writer Julia Blackburn captures the slipperiness of words: "I've often mistrusted the spoken word. You give a quick tug on a line and out they come from the dark continent of the mind, those little rasps of sound that jostle together, shoulder to shoulder, that are supposed to be able to give shape to what you really think, feel, or know. But words easily miss the point. They drift off in the wrong direction, or they insist on providing a clear shape for something that, by its nature, is lost when it's pinned down."

Physics supplies a nice analogy for the principle that each method tells us something different about a phenomenon we wish to understand. The light telescope detects planets and stars, but it can't detect the dark matter that makes up most of the universe. Dark matter is described with a vocabulary different from the one used to describe the information we get from the light telescope.

The descriptions produced by trained introspection are incommensurable with the descriptions obtained from observing behavior or performing a PET scan of a human brain. You cannot translate one set of descriptions into the other. One cannot translate the products of my introspection on how I feel about the war in Iraq into sentences that will describe the fMRI scan of my brain while I'm engaging in the same thoughts in Richard Davidson's laboratory. The physicist Hermann von Helmholtz thought he could describe a Bach fugue with a vocabulary of sine waves and spectra. Brahms, in a conversation with von Helmholtz, disagreed and said he had to use the vocabulary of form, counterpoint, and harmony. We would probably use words like *elegant, aesthetic,* or *relaxing* to describe the fugue. No individual could discover through introspection which area of the brain was more active when she saw a robin fly from a tree and which area was active when she noticed that it had a red breast. No introspection can reveal the subtle distortions we impose on our past experience in the service of creating a coherence that was absent in those experiences.

Finally, and this is very important—I hope it comes up in our discussion—the Buddhist scholars told us that their ethical premises influenced their introspective activity. It is impossible to separate them. That confession means that an individual with a different ethical position will have a different set of introspective experiences about the same event.

I believe, however, that trained introspection can reveal subtleties of perception and feeling that no other current scientific method can discover. That is why I came to this meeting, and this information is useful. I agree with Eric Lander, and the consensus I sense in this meeting, that this evidence should be incorporated into studies of human psychology.

I welcome the contribution of Buddhist scholars to this mission, for they have something important to tell us about the mind and, perhaps, the brain. Although I believe their insights are not more valid—or, if you prefer, more true—than any other empirical corpus, trained introspection remains a valuable source of evidence, another instrument to be added to those of the geneticist, cell biologist, neuroscientist, historian, psychologist, sociologist, anthropologist, novelist, poet, and all who wish to be wiser observers of the phenomena we can never know completely.

With these last remarks, Kagan returned to his seat on the stage. It was now time to see what the group as a whole would have to say. We were a full house. Kagan and Lander were joined by Ajahn Amaro, Alan Wallace, Georges Dreyfus, Evan Thompson, Arthur Zajonc, Jonathan Cohen, Stephen Kosslyn, Richard Davidson, the Dalai Lama, Thupten Jinpa (acting as translator), and Anne Harrington, who took the role of moderator. Together we formed a large and animated semicircle before the audience.

ANNE HARRINGTON: I have now the more or less impossible task of trying, in forty-five minutes, to do justice to all that was put on the table not only in these two very rich, wonderful presentations, but over the past three sessions as well. We are not going to succeed in doing everything. But I envision our having a discussion now that will unfold over time, like a branching tree, from some of the root concerns, the first principles that were eloquently laid out by Jerome Kagan in his remarks. At this level, we must grapple with issues concerning ethics, and the relationship between knowledge and ethics, prescription and description in our two traditions. We may find common ground on these issues, or we may not.

At this level, we also need to discuss questions about epistemology. What kind of status are we hoping to grant to any first-person data offered from the Buddhist side? How do our different understandings of the reliability or status of these kinds of first-person data relate to the status we grant to so-called third-person data—and how do both of those, in turn, relate to truth and to reality?

In his remarks, Eric Lander laid out a set of more concrete questions about the fundamentals needed to carry out constructive collaboration. But we need to know, too: What are the fundamentals in play in terms of the motivations people on both sides bring to their vision of collaboration? What does each side need to understand in that respect, in order for a collaboration to be possible? Once we're clear on that, we can then begin to get practical, roll up our sleeves and get going. We can start then to say, "Okay, what do we want to do? What's next? What's the future? What's the agenda?" Toward the end of our conversation this afternoon, I hope we'll also be able to at least taste some of the possibilities here.

Why don't I begin by inviting His Holiness to speak now to some of the big questions: the relation between ethics and knowledge, the understanding of what introspection is and what we can learn from it, how incorrigible it is or isn't.

DALAI LAMA: One thing that I would like to say is that it would be a mistake to privilege introspection as the key method for examining or investigating the mind, with the implication that anything discovered as a result of such introspective process is valid in some form, somehow reflecting the true nature of things. If we examine our own mental states, including many of the distorted states of mind that wrongly perceive the world, some of them may be more innate, natural, and spontaneous, but many of them are actually based on some form of reasoning. In the Buddhist language we would call them acquired misconceptions. They are acquired as a result of thought processes that are in some sense introspective.

For example, one of the principle premises of Buddhism is the rejection of any form of enduring, intrinsically real self, or soul. From the Buddhist point of view, we would regard those philosophical tenets that uphold the existence of such an eternal principle as intellectually acquired. The way in which they are acquired is seen as a process of introspection or reasoning. People could argue that there is a natural sense of self that we all experience. For example, when we have a visual experience like seeing a flower, the sensory faculties are the instrument that is used to perceive, and therefore we feel there must be something—the thing that experiences the flower—separate from the sensory faculty that does the activity. Since this cannot be identified with the actual senses, it must be some external, transcendental principle. In some cases this kind of introspection can also take the form of meditation.

ARTHUR ZAJONC: I think this question is connected to the whole first-person/third-person way that we handle the introspective observations of Buddhism. But we know from our psychologist friends that introspection also plays an important role within their own disciplines. I wonder if they might speak to this question of the nature of first-person experience and its place in their work; and, vice versa, whether the Buddhists could speak to the importance of third-person experience in their traditions.

ANNE HARRINGTON: As a background comment, we have been feeling that we were at risk here of "giving" the first-person perspective to Buddhism and "giving" the third-person perspective to science. This creates a cartoon of both perspectives, and we have felt it is important that we enrich this picture a little bit.

JONATHAN COHEN: I agree that there is a rich tradition in psychology of attending to the first-person perspective. Perhaps that is best characterized or most fully developed in psychophysics, where there is a tradition of training subjects who attend to percepts that are being studied in the laboratory. At least within that domain, and others as well, first-person reports are a source of data just like any other. They are subject to analysis and to verification with other methods used to measure.

RICHARD DAVIDSON: I want to add one other point regarding the methodology that has been developed in the behavioral sciences for introspection. Not all of it depends on words. Many of us share Jerry Kagan's skepticism and concern about the use of words, and in the tradition of psychophysics, the reports that subjects provide are typically not reports in words. They can scale the intensity of a stimulus using something other than words. An individual might be presented with different intensities of light and be asked to adjust the volume of a sound to be equivalent in intensity to the intensity of the light that they are experiencing. That is an example of using a completely different modality other than words to provide information about experience.

AJAHN AMARO: I think that those who are not used to meditation can make the mistake of assuming that every introspective act is reliable. One of the things His Holiness was referring to is that not everything that runs through our minds, or that we think is intelligent and wise, is necessarily accurate. One of the main elements involved in spiritual training is your relationship with your peers and more particularly with your teacher. If I were to go to my teacher and say, "I'm enlightened! I'm enlightened!" he is probably going to say, "Well, sit down. Let's talk about it."

ALAN WALLACE: I feel a little bit more optimistic about the use of language. If we take an analogy, advanced mathematicians will use coined words that only they understand. They can conceive of the referents of the words, and they are simply speaking a language that I can't. I think the same is true in physics. I share Jerry Kagan's great admiration for Niels Bohr and other people involved in the foundations of quantum mechanics. Bohr, Heisenberg, and others were speaking about things that are simply unimaginable to nonphysicists. Contemporary physics, with its super-string theory of eleven dimensions, is beyond anything I can imagine. And yet, somehow, string theorists are communicating in meaningful ways about things that outsiders cannot even imagine.

Something very similar happens among advanced contemplatives. For example, when for a moment we pause and are simply aware of being aware, what do we find are the salient characteristics of consciousness? Buddhists say, "Clarity and cognizance." But what does "clarity" mean? It's not the same as the clarity of light. It's not clear in the way that any sensory objects are, but it's the best word that we have to indicate what's actually being experienced. The words are being used metaphorically. An outsider, as Ajahn Amaro is suggesting, might not know what contemplatives are talking about or, even worse, mistakenly think they do know what they are talking about, whereas in fact they are interpreting contemplative terminology in terms of everyday experience.

As a translator myself, I'm confident that terminology has been devised among contemplatives so that they can speak in ways that are coherent and revealing among themselves. There's a gradation of how well you might "grok" what they are saying. Having said that, there are also large realms of introspective and contemplative experience about which they will simply say, flat out, "This domain of experience is inconceivable and inexpressible." That's where we stop trying to imagine what they are talking about, because even they can't imagine the referents of their words, though they may experience them directly.

Then what is the use of language? Buddhists use language, as they say, like the finger pointing to the moon. We use language to help us reach a state of realization, ourselves, which, when we get there, is ineffable. But the language will help us get there. Once we think we have gotten there, we come back to Ajahn Amaro's statement. We may think we have achieved some extraordinary state of *samadhi*, or unconditional love, or realization of pure consciousness. That's all very well, but some discussion must then take place between the mentor and the student. Moreover, Buddhism is also pragmatic. It's not just aiming for some ineffable state so we can then walk around proudly thinking we have achieved an ineffable state. If it's an ineffable state that really fathoms the nature of reality, then this should have expression in our behavior in terms of less afflictive or destructive conduct. It should display itself in positive behavior in a myriad of ways. Even though the two languages of first-person experience and third-person observation may be untranslatable in the final analysis, the first-person experience must express itself in observable behavior. And in the domain of the third person, this can be tested by Buddhist techniques as well as scientific.

EVAN THOMPSON: I would like to make a comment about the distinction between first person and third person. We need to be cautious and not fall into too simple a dichotomy. There is actually a plurality of positions and perspectives. We have a first-person singular position in which I, myself, practice the introspection. Then we have a second-person perspective, in which I go to a teacher, a coach, a midwife, or mediator who helps me with the experience. That interaction is linguistically and socially mediated, which means that we are embedded in a first-person plural perspective, an intersubjective context that is essential to any cognitive endeavor, whether contemplative or scientific.

Within that, we have a third-person perspective in which we try to take a critical distance from the observed behavior, whether it's as a clinical or research psychologist, or an anthropologist. Finally, as an asymptotic limit of that, there is what we could call an impersonal perspective, which is the perspective that physics in Western science strives for: the idea of a view from nowhere that in principle has the bias of no particular perspective. Yet it's asymptotic in the sense that the striving for that perspective is always within an intersubjective community. It's a very complex, multifaceted, social situation that we shouldn't lose sight of.

DALAI LAMA: If you examine carefully, whether conclusions are reached through an introspective process based on an individual's own personal experience in observing certain states of the mind, or through empirical observation of external objects, in neither case are the individual's cognitions in a position to determine their own validity. Their validity has to be verified by some other factor. In Buddhist epistemology, we speak of an instance of cognition being valid insofar as it is not contradicted or invalidated by some other third-person observation. This third-person observation could be another individual's observation, or it could be the same individual's cognitive state. For example, it could be a recollection of something or it could be a subsequent cognitive experience. The need for verification from a third person is true in the case of both empirical observation and introspection. In Buddhism, the existence or truth of something is judged on the basis of whether or not there is a valid cognition of that phenomenon. Whether or not the cognition is valid, veridical, or deluded, is determined by another factor.

JONATHAN COHEN: An extension of that point from our side is the use of introspective accounts in studying problem solving. Herb Simon, one of the founders of the field of cognitive science, was very interested in how people use reason to solve problems, and he recognized very early that an important source of information was people's reports of the strategies they were using. He made that a critical source of data, but he didn't stop there. He asked how those reports relate to the measurables, the reaction times that people take for a particular choice that they make. It was the convergent use of both sources of information that provided the most leverage and understanding of the internal processes that people were following.

STEVEN KOSSLYN: The presentation I gave was focused on introspection, so I won't reiterate the main ideas, which were that sometimes introspection does reveal properties of mechanisms and sometimes it doesn't. Something interesting came out of giving that presentation before His Holiness: I discovered that it's not just the introspective reports themselves but the way you elicit them that is crucial. My little demos and trivial questions that worked so well with Harvard undergraduates were not so useful cross-culturally. I think Eric Lander's point about having the Buddhists collaborate in designing the ways we actually elicit the information is crucial. It's a question not just of how we interpret what the reports are but of how we actually design the protocols for getting the information. We need help from you on that as well.

AJAHN AMARO: I'd like to say a little bit about validation in Buddhist practice. I also think it accords very well with the whole spirit of this meeting. There's a very famous teaching in the southern Buddhist scriptures called the Kalama Sutta. The Buddha came through a particular village, and there were many sincere people living there, including spiritual practitioners. They said to the

Buddha, "We get all kinds of gurus and yogis and *sanyasins* and teachers coming through here. Everyone has their own philosophy and everyone says, 'I'm right and all the other guys are wrong.' So we are in doubt as to who we're supposed to believe and what we are supposed to do." The Buddha then said, "You are right to doubt, because you doubt that which should be doubted—because you don't know." Then he gave this very remarkable teaching, where he said, "When you hear something being expressed of this nature, you shouldn't accept it just because it's widespread news that everyone thinks this way. You shouldn't follow it just because it's what your parents do. You shouldn't follow it just because it's the latest new thing. You shouldn't follow it because it's cited in scriptures. You shouldn't follow it because it is hammered out by logic or by inductive or deductive reasoning. And you shouldn't follow it just because it appeals to common sense, or because of the credibility of the speaker, or even because it's your own teacher who's saying it to you." The Buddha then said, "If you take something and apply it, see whether it leads to benefit for yourself and others. Does it make life for yourself more rich, more peaceful, more harmonious, more benevolent? Then take it and use it. If it makes life more difficult and more harmful for yourself and others, then leave it aside." The important point is that validation is also built around a pragmatic outcome. It's not just a matter of establishing truth as an abstract. In the Buddhist method, the individual is certainly the final arbiter of truth, but much weighing and evaluating and experimental examination goes on prior to that.

ARTHUR ZAJONC: Georges Dreyfus spoke about three stages: ethics; *samadhi*, or concentration; and wisdom born of insight into the nature of reality. We have described wisdom in various ways. There are lots of delusions, but there is a reality that we have the possibility of realizing, through all of these methods. I don't think most scientists would make a claim about reality. We could discuss this point.

The second point is that this perception of reality shatters delusions and therefore shatters the sources of attachment. So the Buddhists are making an argument that has a back action. That is to say, this knowledge is transformative. It isn't arms-length knowledge. It isn't knowledge that doesn't change who I am. If I know these things, it has huge possible consequences for me. This is the piece that relates to ethics. This is the essential connection between knowing and transformation, which leads toward enlightenment or liberation. Knowing is part of the project of liberation. That's a very deep statement about the nature of knowledge—a very important statement and a difference, if I'm not mistaken, from our normal scientific understanding of knowing and its implications.

ALAN WALLACE: There is another very bold claim made in Buddhism: that the pursuit of knowledge, if it is to go very, very far, is inextricably related to the pursuit of virtue, and the pursuit of virtue is inextricably related to the pursuit of happiness. When you come to know reality as it is, this experiential insight yields a state of profound and enduring well-being. When you come to know reality as it is, this also spontaneously yields virtues. This is all entangled together. Living a virtuous life will make you more prone to knowing reality as it is, and it will also give rise to greater happiness. Each of these feeds into the others. The pursuit of virtue, including compassion, the pursuit of knowing reality as it is, and the pursuit of genuine happiness are completely integrated. It started that way in the Buddha's own quest and holds true in his teachings ever since then.

This is a notion that we also find in Greek antiquity. We find it in the early centuries of the Christian era. We've almost entirely lost this idea in the present day—that to pursue truth that frees, you must lead a virtuous life. As you succeed in this, it will give rise to happiness and a profound state of well-being. Although we may have lost this, I don't think it's entirely alien to our civilization. We have suffered some amnesia.

JEROME KAGAN: That's said so beautifully and elegantly that you can see the contrast: that is not the view of Western science. I mean this with no evaluation, but I think that's why the audience is applauding. We can have an absolutely amoral scientist discovering a beautiful truth about nature. That's a problem. The use of the word *knowledge* is slipping around here, as in Julia Blackburn's quote. We are using it in different ways, and so we have to be very careful.

MATTHIEU RICARD: It seems that there is a very big distance between ethics and knowing reality. When we speak of knowing reality properly, it doesn't mean that we will correctly evaluate the size of something or will not be fooled by an optical illusion. What we mean by the nature of reality is precisely those things that it matters to know in a certain way in order to get rid of suffering. For instance, if we grasp at something as being permanent though it is not—it is transitory, changing every moment—when we lose it, we are going to suffer. We innately equate things that we believe are permanent with reality. In the same way, we believe that things have intrinsic properties. We believe that something is 100 percent beautiful in itself and therefore we need to get it; we strive for it. We have an improper perception of the reality of interdependent phenomena, which are mainly relations between the subject and the object. All phenomena are just a stream of constant transformation. If we don't see it like that, then we are at odds with reality. An improper perception of this nature of the phenomenal world will lead to a wrong perception of the phenomenal world in terms of desire and rejection, and will end up in a sense of frustration and suffering.

In that sense, ethics in the Buddhist perspective are not commandments from the outside, are not abstract or absolute ideas, like Platonic ideas. Buddhist ethics are intimately linked with the law of cause and effect in terms of happiness and suffering. A wrong perception of reality is also closely linked with ethics as a science of the mechanism of well-being and suffering. The way we perceive the world has a connection with the way we behave, the way we experience happiness and suffering, and the way we bring it to others.

DALAI LAMA: We are throwing this word *ethics* around. From my point of view, ethics have to be tied to the basic fact of our experience of pain and happiness. We don't desire suffering, and we always aspire to be free of suffering. Restraint from the conditions that lead to suffering is ethics. It is very difficult to judge the ethicality of an act purely from the point of view of the act itself, given the complexity of the context in which our actions come into being. For example, we can imagine a particular act that may be harmful in a very specific context. If you indulge in that act in that context, it is unethical. However, in a totally different context, not engaging in that very same act may lead to suffering. So it is very difficult to determine ethicality objectively. The ethicality of an act has to be understood in relation to its conditions for giving rise to either suffering or happiness. A further complexity with suffering and happiness is that we have to take into account the long-term and short-term perspectives, and the benefit for a single individual or for a larger group.

JONATHAN COHEN: This is an absolutely essential issue, and I'm really glad we've gotten to it. Anne mentioned a few minutes ago that from the Western perspective there is a separation, much like the separation of church and state, between scientific results and ethicality. Before I say more, I want to make it really clear that we are talking about the results of science, not the practice of science. Nobody disputes that scientists should do their best to abide by a code of ethics and morality in their pursuit of science. The question is whether the results of science have prescriptive status for ethics, or are simply descriptive.

My personal belief—and I will be eager to hear what my colleagues have to say—is that that separation of church and state is a luxury tied to the fact that science has for so long focused primarily on the external and not the internal. If we take a pragmatist's view of ethics, as described here, and we say that ethics concerns internal states and suffering, and if we now extend science to the study of those internal states through psychology and neuroscience, it may be that science no longer has the luxury of remaining separate from ethics.

As we learn about suffering—the conditions that produce suffering over the short or long term, that produce local or global suffering—and the processes that give rise to ethical decisions, and the consequences of those decisions, we may have to confront the possibility that science will soon have something to say about the prescription of ethics and not just continue to assume a purely descriptive stance.

JEROME KAGAN: I think Eric made a very important point when he said, "The facts of science are only one avenue of truth." The problem in our society, and a reason why many of you are applauding selectively, is that humans want or need a source of support for their moral beliefs. Science has become the moral arbiter in Western society. But some true facts about nature bother our ethics; for example, *Homo sapiens* is, as a matter of fact, a sexually promiscuous species. Should we change our laws? Of course not. That's why you, members of the public, are not being foolish or dumb when you say to the scientists, "Mr. and Mrs. Scientist, that is a very interesting fact that you've discovered, but I choose not to implement policy based on it." It would be terrible if we felt we had to act on every scientific fact because it was a true description of nature. Many people have understood this before. We evolved with this ethical sense. That is the deep Buddhist understanding. And it's a totally unique thing in evolution. It allows us to decide whether a practice is something we wish to take up or not, based on our deep ethical sense, and some of our choices can be inconsistent with what is true about nature!

ALAN WALLACE: I'd like to raise a scientific and empirical question: Is there such a thing as genuine happiness? We need to define genuine happiness. I'm not talking in abstract terms; rather, I am speaking of a state of well-being that is inspired by the ancient Greek notion of *eudaimonia*, a sense of human flourishing that carries us through times of adversity and felicity, in times of sickness and good health, all the vicissitudes of daily life. Is there such a thing? How do we define it? This assumes we could define it—as you can define a tachyon, for example, before ever finding one—and then see if there is any empirical evidence for it. Can you find people whose behavior, the way they live in the world and speak and act, suggests that they have found at least some degree of *eudaimonia*, or genuine happiness?

If you can define it and find empirical evidence for it, then you can ask further scientific questions. What modes of life are conducive to yielding genuine happiness? There are situations that are not at all unpleasant in which people find themselves clinically depressed. There are situations that are not at all adverse in which people are terribly angry. They generate these emotions internally. If there is such a thing as genuine happiness, then define it, find empirical evidence for it, and then study it scientifically and empirically to see what modes of life, what attitudes, what qualities of attention, emotion, and so forth, are conducive to it. Similarly, find what modes of behavior, attitudes, or mental activities yield unnecessary suffering. Turn that into a science. Why not?

JEROME KAGAN: Because I don't believe there is one unitary "happiness." There are many, many happinesses, and each one has different qualia. Therefore we have to look for a multitude family.

ALAN WALLACE: Indeed. Why not look for a multitude family?

ANNE HARRINGTON: Eric Lander gave us a wonderfully eloquent set of preconditions for moving forward in a partnership of mutually respectful collaboration. I suggest that we focus on his question: What are the most fruitful areas of collaboration? Where do we go from here? What, specifically, from both sides, would you most desire to have happen next?

JONATHAN COHEN: I don't want this to sound glib, but I feel like there's a figure-ground shift that could be made in some of the discussion about experiments. We keep thinking about the Buddhists as the object of study, comparing them and their unique abilities with what we might consider normal. We ask how they excel, and the notion that they may excel in certain important ways is intriguing. But if we take their statements at face value, which I am certainly eager to do, and believe that they have a means of achieving a state of normality—where normality means normalization of a kind of equanimity of emotion and spirit—then in some sense that should be the baseline condition. Experiments might be designed to see how we differ from that state. If there's a truth to the claim, we should be able to define differences that map onto forms of suffering that we can identify, as well. This strikes me as one possible way of reconfiguring our thinking about how to do experiments.

AJAHN AMARO: When Jonathan and I were talking about this the other day, I suggested that perhaps we could invite the psychologists to a ten-day retreat.

JONATHAN COHEN: And I went white!

GEORGES DREYFUS: Rather than defining particular research projects, this meeting has been very interesting for me in our trying to define the conceptual terms as well as the ethical conditions for fruitful collaboration. That has been so revealing. I think we have made quite a lot of progress in understanding what is involved in that collaboration, what the pitfalls are, the terms on which fruitful collaboration can be based, and, obviously, some of the ethical dimensions of that collaboration. So far as particular projects are concerned, it breaks down into what a particular researcher or group wants to do.

ERIC LANDER: I would like to emphasize the importance of the point that the Buddhists may be better able to tell us what kinds of psychological and psychophysical tests one would apply to capture whether someone has or has not attained an ability to attend or to control emotion. I would like to push the point, because some of those tests can be done without the MRIs in Wisconsin. They could be done by Buddhists in Dharamsala. For a meaningful research collaboration to go on, it must go on in India and Tibet as well. It's just good science. We must both actually be engaged in designing experiments to have the best conversation. A great outcome would be Tibetan Buddhists doing and publishing experiments with colleagues in these countries in the next few years. That's something demonstrable one could try to accomplish. I think they would be different experiments than would otherwise be conceived, and very interesting. The experiments could get picked up and then replicated in the West.

MATTHIEU RICARD: After two or three years, now, of collaboration, I would frame our perspective in a simple way. It comes from our intimate conviction that we have found the training we have been through to be extremely useful, if not precious, in terms of personal transformation and well-being. Of course we know we have traits and predispositions, but our belief is that transformation came through the training; that is our assumption. So it would be interesting to have some clues from the results of testing individuals who have gone through this training. If we find some differences, that is already an indication that there is something worthy there. I completely agree that the main point now will be to validate the notion of mind training by taking individuals who have not yet engaged in this training, or are midway through it, and testing them over time. I think that is the main point. If it's true that we are born with that skill because of our genes or environment, and that those traits are immutable, then we have just chosen the right life to enjoy what we are and there's not much that we can contribute to others. But if it's true that I wasn't at all like this when I was at the Pasteur Institute, and that the benefit I have derived comes from a combination of skillful and wonderfully compassionate and wise teachers along with my own efforts in this training—if that is true, as I'm personally convinced—then that's what I want to contribute to humankind. In that sense, investigating the process of transformation would be the most useful program of research. It will take time, but it is the most valid approach.

ANNE HARRINGTON: In our decision here to pay particular attention to the Buddhist contemplative tradition and what it can reveal about the workings or trainability of the mind, we face both a question and a potential misunderstanding: Are we in fact inviting an understanding of Buddhism as a privileged contemplative tradition—and as the only means by which one can gain greater self-control or balance? I wonder if anyone wants to speak to that.

AJAHN AMARO: Certainly the Buddhists would not claim to have a monopoly on mind training or on skillful qualities in any way. There is a passage in our scriptures where someone asks the Buddha, "Is the path that you describe the only way to freedom, to fulfillment as a human being?" And he says, "No. I happen to articulate it in this way, but it is not the only way. Any form of training will do, as long as it contains *sila*, the ethical element; mind training in concentration and mental focus; mental stability or *samadhi*; and training in the wisdom of insight—not just wisdom in terms of acquisition of knowledge, information, and ideas, but a deep insight into the fundamental nature of reality as a direct experience. As long as the teaching contains those elements, it can certainly lead any human being to full realization of the true nature of things. The language, the imagery and symbolism in which one casts those principles, is secondary.

RICHARD DAVIDSON: I wanted to follow up on Eric Lander's comment, which is extremely important. We are at the stage now, for those interested in collaboration, where we can begin to think about exporting or inventing behavioral tasks in another culture.

One of the wonderful side products of doing collaborative research of this kind, as laboratory scientists know, is that there's an awful lot of dead time in the lab when you're not actually collecting data. During those times, conversations have taken place in which germinal ideas for new designs and new tasks to better capture the impact of the mental training have been discussed. That is a very hopeful consequence of this collaboration, and I think we will see the products of that in the future.

AJAHN AMARO: I wanted to underscore something that Jerry Kagan said in his wonderful address. He outlined very clearly how extraordinarily difficult it is to put into words some of these subtle

realities and experiences. I just want to reassure you that at first
even the Buddha didn't think it was worth trying. He had to be
persuaded.

*We wrapped up the conversation at this point, because we had agreed
in advance that the Dalai Lama would have the last word, and that
his final remarks would be addressed not to the scholars and scientists
on stage, but to the audience. At the invitation of Anne Harrington, he
rose to his feet and went to the podium. His translator, Thupten Jinpa,
accompanied him, since, when it is important to him to make himself
precisely understood, he usually chooses to speak in Tibetan. What
follows is Thupten Jinpa's on-the-spot translation of the Dalai Lama's
closing comments.*

DALAI LAMA: I have been able to participate in these two days of
conversations with the scientists and fellow Buddhist scholars. Although my own command of English is not adequate to be able to
follow all the exchanges, I was still able to follow quite a lot with
the patchy English that I have. It has made me feel really refreshed, alert, and also joyful. As I listened to the presentations of
Eric Lander and Jerome Kagan, who made a beautiful summation
of some of the salient points that were raised in the conversations,
I felt deeply impressed, and the only thing I could say is, yes, I
agree with you. Today I really felt like being a Yes Minister. I
would also like to take the opportunity to express my thanks to all
the speakers who made beautiful presentations in a very lucid and
succinct form with such confidence and knowledge. My own intuition for the possibility of benefits through conversations between
Buddhism and science goes back quite a long time, but every time
I have had the opportunity to participate in one of these conversations, my enthusiasm for such conversations increases. One of the
consequences of participating in these dialogues is that every time,
as I approach the end of the discussions, I have an enthusiastic desire to learn more English. Then after a few months it passes, and

my English never progresses. In fact, as I get older, my English also gets older.

One of the facts of our modern society is that many people have faith and confidence in science, as well as an admiration for science. This admiration and faith in science really should not be diminished by any fear that science might bring about disaster or crisis. Basically, science is one way to bring more happiness to humanity. Of course, sometimes, technology brings a few negative consequences. That is not necessarily because there is something wrong with science and technology; it comes from the wrong ways that we human beings use these things. Ultimately the mistake is our own. Science itself is wonderful, something of service to humanity.

Buddhism, like any other religion, has always taught compassion, loving-kindness, forgiveness, tolerance, contentment, and self-discipline. These are very useful in order to have happy days and nights. All religions talk about them the same way, so all have the same potential to help humanity. Buddhism advocates the cultivation of compassion for human beings but also extends it to infinite sentient beings, not just for one lifetime but through infinite lives. Buddhism's basic aim is to help and serve sentient beings.

Science until now has mainly dealt with external physical things, and generally Buddhism, like other spiritual traditions, deals primarily with internal values. We human beings have a physical body, but we also have this mind. To have a happy, meaningful life, we have to take care of our body as well as our mind. So I think spiritual traditions and material progress should go together, in combination.

In the Buddhist contemplative tradition, right from its earliest inception, the importance of investigating the nature of reality has been a very central point. If you look at the Buddha's own teachings on the Four Noble Truths—the truth of suffering, the truth of its origin, the truth of the cessation of suffering, and the path to that cessation—we find a presentation of these four truths from the perspective of the specific nature of suffering, its origins and so on, which pertains to understanding the nature of reality. There is also a description of these Four Noble Truths from the point of view of their functions, which concern the ethical actions that one must engage in on the basis of understanding reality. The third perspective that the Buddha brings is the result of such ethical activity, which the Buddhist language refers to as the fruition of the spiritual path.

The Buddhist contemplative teachings are always presented within this framework of understanding the nature of reality, the path—ethical actions based on reality, and the fruition or result of the spiritual path. In the teachings of the Buddha himself, there is a recognition that the quality of the results that you experience is contingent on the causes and the conditions that give rise to it. When cultivating the understanding of the nature of reality, Buddhism speaks of avoiding two forms of wrong views. One is the wrong view based on exaggeration or reification: one exaggerates and superimposes qualities and characteristics over and above what is there in actual reality. The other wrong view is described as the wrong view of denigration, where you in fact denigrate and subtract from what is actually already there in phenomena. To cultivate the right view, one must avoid falling into these two extremes. Here we see again the emphasis placed on encouraging the understanding of reality.

One could say that, broadly speaking, science is also engaged in the pursuit of understanding reality. In that sense, at least in terms of spirit, there is a commonality between Buddhism and science.

To return to the question of ethics based on this understanding of reality, we can ask: Can one make sense of any discussion of ethical concepts before the origination of human beings? Probably not. From the Buddhist point of view, the understanding of ethics must be tied to the human quest for the fulfillment of our basic aspiration, which is to overcome suffering and achieve happiness. Returning to the Buddha's original teaching of the Four Noble

Truths on suffering and its causes, the Buddha taught that we must overcome the causes of suffering, and cultivate the path that leads to the cessation of suffering. The basic idea of ethics is already presented—refraining from negative actions and engaging in virtuous actions. This is directly tied to our basic project of overcoming suffering and seeking happiness.

I think, generally speaking, scientific research also tries to investigate matters that may have some benefit for us: harmful things, which we try to eliminate, and positive things we try to increase. How do we do that? I think the answer is to know the nature of the reality, and how opposing forces counter each other. So, for example, if a particular force is harmful, we have to find its opposing force. We can then enhance one and help diminish the other.

It is exactly the same in the inner world. Some emotions are beneficial and some emotions, such as hatred, are harmful. How do we reduce hatred? We have to find out what the opposing force is and apply it. That opposition will help reduce it. This is again related to the basic understanding of certain laws of nature—that there are certain opposing forces in the natural world, where if you strengthen one side, it has the corresponding effect of reducing the force of the other.

Of course I am not here to preach Buddhadharma. *(laughter)* On the panel, we were talking about a very important issue: How to move forward? What collaborative projects can we envision through this joint conversation? A lot of suggestions have been made. My own feeling is that we should not confine this vision to our own generation alone. It has to be thought through in terms of a long-term vision so that it can go beyond our generation.

I think we need better education for the mind: more sophisticated minds to match more sophisticated technology. With the present situation, if we do not pay sufficient attention to the inner emotional world, there is a danger. All this technology can be used for negative purposes. Look at what happened in 2001, on September 11. This makes the point very clearly.

Scientists also have emotions, just like I do. Buddhists are full of emotion. As human beings, Buddhists, too, get into a lot of trouble because of some of these emotions. You are similar. As long as we are human beings, we have these emotions. Our experiences are the same. Do not consider this as a religious matter but simply as one method of knowing what are the positive emotions and then trying to encourage those emotions and discourage negative emotions. As a result, you will be happier and calmer. I think you could carry on your scientific research more effectively that way. If your mind holds much disturbance, your mental agitation may cause you to do some wrong things.

This is what I usually call secular ethics. It has nothing to do with religion. Christianity, Judaism, Islam, and Hinduism talk about God, heaven, and such things. Buddhism, too, also talks about the next life and nirvana, and so on. In the context of what I call secular ethics, we can forget about these things. Our aim is simply to try to be a better human being.

So that's our goal. As long as human beings remain on this planet, this is our work and we'll continue. Thank you.

ARTHUR ZAJONC

Reflections on "Investigating the Mind," One Year Later

CHAPTER NINE

Introspective observation is what we have to rely on first and foremost and always.
—William James

At the opening of "Investigating the Mind," the eleventh Mind and Life meeting (ML XI), Evan Thompson challenged us to move beyond the "taboo of subjectivity" and to engage the phenomenology of consciousness with a sophistication that has, in his view, been absent from research in cognitive science. While scientists traditionally use naive subjects and ask them to report verbally and otherwise on their mental states, he said that a much richer and more rigorous first-person methodology should be developed and joined to the well-developed third-person research methods already practiced. Thompson suggested that the persistent pursuit of the neural correlates of consciousness should give way to a more balanced and integrated approach in which *experience* has as important a role in consciousness research as neural mechanisms. In his appeal on behalf of experience he invoked the legacy of William James, whose seminal work on the mind proved to be a touchstone for many throughout the meeting. The other scientific lineage invoked by Thompson was that of Francisco Varela. Varela coined the term *neurophenomenology* to convey a vision of a research methodology in which neuroscience, phenomenological observation, and meditative schooling would in the future be joined together to provide a foundation for consciousness research.

As this volume testifies, Thompson's challenge to speak from experience was amply met by the Buddhist scholar-practitioners. They offered detailed descriptions of both the path of contemplative cultivation and the results of attentive introspective observation. At the conference, we learned how expert meditators, in place of untrained, naive subjects, were taking on a new role as collaborators with their scientific colleagues. We also learned that, in addition to their developed contemplative skills, Buddhist scholars possess a sophisticated philosophical and theoretical framework for thinking about mental experience. Although the Buddhists could say little about questions concerning mechanism, their nuanced taxonomies of the inner life and their apparent ability to maintain sustained control of their mental state challenged certain fundamental assumptions of Western cognitive science. In the spirit of open-minded inquiry, the scientists at the meeting welcomed the opportunity to test such claims experimentally. Many were excited about the possibility that they were witnessing something genuinely new: a new kind of science dealing with an enormously important area—the mind.

To help assess the impact of the two-day meeting, I asked speakers, panelists, and some attendees for their reflections, positive and critical. I have woven their responses through the following pages to provide views of the gathering from varied perspectives.

Orthogonal Views

In cross-cultural discussions, we quickly become aware that our so-called facts are theory laden. The very way we parse the data on the mental life reflects our unspoken presuppositions and aims. Even with goodwill on both sides, this became strikingly evident in the ML XI meeting at MIT—and nowhere more powerfully than in the contrasting treatments of emotion in Buddhist psychology and affective cognitive psychology. The Buddhist scholar Georges Dreyfus reminded us that there is no word for emotion in Tibetan, and that the Abhidharma's extensive taxonomy of mental life mingles emotions with nonemotional factors such as ignorance and laziness. Neuroscientist Richard Davidson's account, in contrast, described a two-dimensional matrix of emotion with valence (pleasant to unpleasant) on one axis and the intensity of the feeling on the other. In this system all emotions are mapped onto the plane formed by these intersecting axes. The differences between the approaches could hardly have been more dramatic. As Eric Lander commented in our final dialogue session: "Their taxonomies differ. They're probably both wrong at some level. Nonetheless, the fact that you have two approaches that don't map onto each other is very valuable."

Lander's point was that it is precisely where two traditions are no longer on common ground that we probably have the most to learn. As Richard Davidson noted, the classification of emotions in the West has been largely shaped by our interest in the body and in behavior. In Buddhism the taxonomies have been formed by more spiritual concerns. Dreyfus emphasized that the search for enlightenment (understood as freedom from afflictions) was a crucial determining factor in shaping the way the Abhidharma organizes practices and knowledge. This orientation may well imply that not all of the Abhidharma's fifty-one mental factors have bodily correlates.

In consequence, while the Abhidharma's detailed description of the inner life greatly intrigued some of the Western scientists, for others it did not address the issues at the level they found most interesting. For example, after participating in the meeting Anne Treisman of Princeton wrote,

What I found least helpful were the lists of categories, of states, the fine distinctions, which for me don't map onto my experience. That would also be true, actually, if the lists came from a Western religion or philosophy. I don't think at that level or type of abstraction. I like to have concrete statements or claims or interpretations about what is happening, with examples, and if possible with some reference to possible mechanisms, either psychological or neural. It is simply a different way of thinking that doesn't answer the kinds of questions I want to ask.

The Buddhists' nuanced distinctions among mental states was matched by complex descriptions of the practices used to control attention, mental imagery, and emotions. As Matthieu Ricard described the traditions for developing mental imagery, we learned that the practice can involve visualizing hundreds of deities and their myriad attributes. The Dalai Lama also provided a meticulous analysis of the forms of attention and the schooling for them. Among the scientists and the audience, admiration for the depth of learning and practice involved was palpable. Following Ricard's presentation, Stephen Kosslyn was warmly applauded when he remarked that "learning about these observations should remind us how little we in the scientific community know about imagery, just how narrow and focused we've been . . . We hope that we are starting to make a few bricks that can contribute to the wall, but we really must be modest in any claims we make at this very early stage of our development."

Scientists come to participate in meetings with the Dalai Lama for many reasons, some purely scientific and others more personal. Few come with a comprehensive understanding of Tibetan Buddhism, and most assume that Western science is in possession of a far more detailed and sophisticated knowledge of the mind. Like star athletes, Buddhists may be great meditators, but they are presumed to have primitive notions of mental life and its cultivation. When the scientists meet the Dalai Lama and other Buddhist scholar-practitioners, however, they soon discover the erudition of their counterparts and the sophistication of their philosophical views. Buddhist empirical claims are situated within genuine theoretical considerations. In Jonathan Cohen's words, "The most gratifying part of this experience is disabusing ourselves of that narrowness of mind and realizing that there are some very interesting ideas that stand behind the claims."

With this realization, Western scientists discover that in Buddhist scholars they have true colleagues. They then turn the table and begin to seek ways to help Buddhist scholar-practitioners with their own research into the mind. At the conference, Nancy Kanwisher of MIT, among others, suggested that simple behavioral experiments would be possible that could help monks check their attentional stability and other mental functions. Jonathan Cohen was applauded when he said to the monks: "I can think of a million things to measure, but I'm interested in what *you* think would be the right things to measure. That would instruct us as much in our perspective as it would allow us to understand yours better."

In a conversation with Thupten Jinpa after the ML XI meeting, I asked him about the significance of such research for the monastic community in India. He replied that it could be quite important. Although the Dalai Lama is enthusiastic about collaborating with scientists, many other Tibetan teachers are primarily concerned with preserving the cultural and spiritual traditions of Tibet while they are in exile. They are therefore quite understandably skittish about teaching Western secular science. If, however, they could become more directly involved in research that assisted them in their own project of cultivating the mind, Jinpa felt this would be a great stimulus for them to include science in their monastic school curriculum.[1]

As discussed in the introduction to this volume, until the meeting at MIT, the Mind and Life dialogues between scientists and the Dalai Lama had taken place in an intimate setting with no real public audience. This time the exchanges were very public, with more than 1,000 people in attendance, primarily from the academic community. Harvard psychologist Daniel Gilbert observed an ironic dynamic that arose in consequence of this; one that he viewed as problematic. As he described it after the conference:

> What could have been a constructive dialogue became a bit of a "gotcha" session in which science was cast as an arrogant and my-opic enterprise that had somehow overlooked the importance of subjective experience, when in fact many areas of modern psychology (for example, mine!) are attempts to study subjective experience with objective methods. I don't think the monks or His Holiness the Dalai Lama were responsible for this unfortunate dynamic. Rather, I fear the scientists may have created it by behaving in an uncharacteristically contrite and self-deprecating manner. The audience ate it up and egged them on with applause that came uncomfortably close to "keeping score." Perhaps the scientists' reverence for His Holiness was incompatible with their typical style of argument and debate. Alas, respect has a place in the quest for truth, but reverence does not. The meeting would have been more useful if it had been more irreverent.

If some perceived audience responses to the presentations as partisan, others felt they simply reflected a collective emotional engagement in what many saw as a historic event. And for some participants, at least, the activities on stage were more than academic—they stimulated deep reflection on personal life choices. I received, for example, this response from Claus Otto Scharmer, a social change theorist at MIT: "When I left this two-day session I saw with the utmost clarity what was wrong with my current life: I was busy with a zillion projects in a zillion places—no focus. With the same clarity, I saw what I should be doing for the years to come: focusing all my activities on a disciplined investigation of the triangle between science, spirituality, and social change. Science and spirituality were at issue on both of the days. But how they relate to the third element, social change, seems to me the call and question of our time."

Returning to the theme of orthogonality, a significant difference between science and Buddhism showed up in the emphasis placed by modern science on the causal relationship between biological evolution and specific attributes of the mind. In the Western scientific tradition, anger, fear, visual perception, and the like are all understood as products of evolution, with the traits in question having features that enhanced genetic fitness in the evolution of the species. As Georges Dreyfus pointed out, Buddhism has little to contribute to the evolutionary interpretation of the origins of fear or anger. It is concerned, rather, with the ways in which these emotions affect us in our own time. How do we spontaneously respond to the arousal of fear, lust, hatred, greed, jealousy, and so on? Do they set in motion a series of unreflective reactions that propel us on a determined course of action? Is it not possible to become aware of them and their destructive or constructive place in the mind, and so control them? In what measure are we free or unfree in relation to these powerful emotions? The Buddhists consistently spoke of a meta-level of awareness that can assess the varied states or experience of consciousness. This level of awareness is essential to judging the quality of mental stability and sensing emotional imbalance. One must know when imbalance prevails in order to redress it. In this view, one is born not free but with the potential to become free. The path of meditative schooling is a long path to freedom, as Alan Wallace stated, which the Buddhist terms enlightenment or liberation.

From conversation with Thupten Jinpa, I know that the Dalai Lama was pleased that a rapport quickly developed at the ML XI meeting that allowed discussion not only of specific Buddhist empirical claims but also of larger philosophical — epistemological and ethical — issues. After the meeting, in response to my queries, many scientists and Buddhists said they would have liked an opportunity to move beyond the preliminary exchanges to a fuller exploration of the important questions raised. For example, in reflecting back on the conference a year later, the philosopher Evan Thompson posed the question: What will scientists accept as a valid science of the mind, and how open are they, really, to a full inclusion of the first-person perspective? He wrote:

In the case of the scientists, I felt the need for a more critical, epistemological perspective on what a science of the mind is or can be. For example, is the scientific interest in Buddhism motivated by wanting to uncover more detailed neural correlates and mechanisms of imagery, attention, and so on? Is a science of the mind ultimately no more than a science of the brain at various levels of abstraction (physiological, functional, etc.), seen as a third-person biological object? Or will a full science of the mind necessarily have an ineliminable first-person, phenomenological component?

Criteria for Collaboration

In his summary remarks at the close of ML XI, Eric Lander described what he saw as the preconditions for collaboration between science and Buddhism or any similar tradition. His first criterion was openness, which, in my judgment, the Buddhists and scientists at the MIT conference amply achieved. The participants' respect for and interest in the views and claims of their counterparts were clear throughout the meeting—something one might not have expected, especially from the perspective of a religious tradition. Buddhism, at least as practiced by the Dalai Lama, seems to value direct experience and reason above revelation and faith, thereby creating an unusual opportunity for dialogue and collaboration. On prior occasions the Dalai Lama has stated his willingness to set aside established Buddhist doctrine if compelling empirical evidence is offered by science. However, he is also aware that sometimes scientists make poorly grounded assertions, oversimplify, and speculate without sufficient evidence to support their claims. In longer meetings he has been a sharp debating partner, probing the limits of empirically based statements and homing in on what he has perceived to be inadequately supported claims.

What features would be required of a contemplative or spiritual philosophy to allow a fruitful collaboration with science? Commitment to experience and reason must certainly rate high, whereas severe barriers would arise if dogmatic theological positions were held. I do not view Tibetan Buddhism as uniquely suited to such a collaboration, but it does evidence the qualities we would need to have for any deep exchange. Perhaps the more contemplative (that is, experiential) and philosophically oriented spiritual traditions within Western Judaism and Christianity could offer a comparable basis for exchange.

We are all familiar with the importance of experimentation in the scientific tradition. Experimentation allows for the systematic control of all factors that might affect an outcome, and for the isolation of the effect under study. Less familiar to us are the efforts made by Buddhist practitioners to develop a parallel set of introspective methods that would permit a detailed exploration of the mind. In this sense, the two traditions both place a high value on controlled empirical exploration, but the directions of those explorations have been quite different. The traditions also both recognize the importance of verification or falsification. The Dalai Lama spoke in particular about how meditative experience should be supported by other factors, such as reason, intersubjective agreement, or traditional authority. Corroboration within a community of scholar-practitioners is important if one is not to be caught by errors in one's personal introspective cognition. Such cautions are sensible, and they are an important indicator of further parallels between Buddhist contemplative research methods and the research methods practiced within the scientific community. Lander cited these considerations in pointing out that the ML XI meeting had not been a "flight from science." Quite the contrary, it had been an extension of scientific discourse to include perspectives that, while foreign to the scientific tradition, were not antithetical to its methods.

All the participants recognized that the greatest difference between the two traditions concerned their focus. In his opening and closing remarks, the Dalai Lama expressed admiration for the great achievements of the sciences, particularly the physical sciences. Buddhism has nothing comparable. He said, however, that Buddhism possesses complementary strengths based on its centuries of research into the mind. Building on the philosophies and contemplative traditions of ancient India, and on the Nalanda University tradition in particular, the Dalai Lama suggested that Tibetan Buddhism can offer important insights into the character and schooling of the mind. Psychology is a relatively young science in the West, and he maintained that Buddhism's long experience could perhaps contribute to this important area of research.

Francisco Varela's original hope for the Mind and Life dialogues was to extend science in exactly this way. The first fruits of including results from highly trained, first-person introspection in cognitive science were in evidence at the ML XI meeting. By the end of the conference, both sides showed growing optimism that the project was doable. Even Jerome Kagan, one of the more cautious and skeptical commentators at the meeting, was convinced and said, "I agree with Eric Lander and the consensus in this meeting, that that evidence [from trained introspection] should be incorporated into our studies of human psychology." William James's emphasis on experience was reaffirmed, and the abiding skepticism against introspection within the psychological community was decisively countered. The most difficult part remained, however: sustained collaboration directed toward establishing the research practices of the emerging field Varela called neurophenomenology.

Genuine research partnerships that draw on the best of Buddhism and the best of science presuppose a common goal or project in which the partners are equals. It would seem important, then, that at least some Buddhist practitioners should be sufficiently familiar with Western scientific protocols that they could become partners in devising the experimental design. Contemplatives have the most intimate knowledge of the phenomena to be studied. It is therefore reasonable to expect that they should be an invaluable resource in experimental design, if one can presume some level of competency in Western science. Partnerships should not be limited to experimental design, however, but should include more theoretical consideration, a point made by both Richard Davidson and Jonathan Cohen at the ML XI meeting. Some parts of the theory of mind offered by Buddhism may well be amenable to confirmation, refinement, or falsification by Western research methods. Finally, as suggested by a number of the scientists, the Buddhists themselves may one day become active researchers in their own communities, using relatively simple behavior research methods and reporting their findings in journals of science. The picture that emerged at the conference was one of two traditions that might learn from each other on several levels: methodological, theoretical, philosophical, and ethical.

In a private communication one year after the ML XI meeting, I asked neuroscientist Richard Davidson what he felt the meeting had accomplished. He responded:

I found the event itself to be useful and historic because it conveyed to a wide scientific audience the potential utility of this dialogue. A major thrust of this meeting was the suggestion that cognitive and emotional processes that have heretofore been regarded as relatively fixed and immutable may be subject to training and improvement through rigorous mind training. Such training can occur because of the known plasticity of the brain. These observations form the basis for unusual possible collaborations and for a mechanistic understanding of how mind training can produce changes in cognitive and affective function.

Evan Thompson expressed Varela's hope for the future in these words, "Francisco's vision, in its boldest and most provocative form, was that future cognitive neuroscientists would be trained in contemplative phenomenology as well as brain-imaging techniques and mathematical modeling; at the same time, contemplative phenom-enologists would be knowledgeable in neuroscience and experimen-tal psychology. The two perspectives would mutually constrain and enrich each other, and would hybridize into the rich science of men-tal life James originally envisioned." Although the ML XI meeting did not realize Varela's vision, one could sense an interest in developing this vision, and even see ways in which people were taking first steps toward its fulfillment.

Research

The most promising example in this context was that offered by Rich-ard Davidson and his collaborator Matthieu Ricard. The unique biog-raphies of both researchers were important for the success of their col-laboration and should be borne in mind when envisioning future collaborations. Prior to becoming a Tibetan monk and a student of meditation more than thirty years ago, Ricard earned his Ph.D. in cell genetics at the Institut Pasteur in Paris. He thus embodies the rare combination of competencies imagined by Varela: scientific school-ing and long contemplative training. Likewise, Richard Davidson is an authority on the neuroscience of emotions and simultaneously has a long-standing interest in meditation. As a graduate student he took a leave of absence to travel through India and Sri Lanka in order to study Asian contemplative techniques.

Together with Antoine Lutz from Varela's lab in Paris, Davidson and Ricard carried out a set of landmark experiments using expert Buddhist meditators as subjects. The first results were published in 2004 in the *Proceedings of the National Academy of Sciences*.[2] The study showed that long-term Buddhist practitioners were able to self-induce sustained electroencephalographic gamma-band oscillations and phase synchrony during meditation. These oscillations were the highest reported in the literature. The investigators interpreted these results as supporting the view that attention and affective processes can be trained. Davidson, Lutz, and Ricard will continue their collab-oration at the Keck Laboratory for Functional Brain Imaging and Behavior at the University of Wisconsin, and we can expect further results from the group in the coming years.

Although research on meditation already has a long history, with thousands of papers published on the subject, the field appears poised to take a new step in its development.[3] If Davidson, Lutz, and Ricard's results are replicated, and if measurements of other mental faculties show comparable improvement with extended meditative practice, then the field of cognitive science will need to revise its theoretical models of mental function and trainability to accommodate these findings. Conversely, if the results of further experiments disconfirm the literature and practice of Buddhist meditators, they will need to moderate their claims accordingly. In either case, informative results can be expected. In a private communication about the conference, Buddhist scholar-practitioner Alan Wallace put it this way: "The Buddhists were short on data. As Eric Lander rightly pointed out in his closing comments, the Buddhists in this meeting made a great many claims that either contradict or transcend current scientific understanding of the mind. But they don't have compelling objective data to back up these claims. The time is now ripe to conduct rigorous scientific research on a wide range of meditative disciplines to determine whether they do in fact yield the types of benefits that have been ascribed to them."

Related to research, Evan Thompson was concerned about the basis and character of the Buddhist claims at ML XI. He wrote to me about this, saying:

In the case of the Buddhists, I felt the need for a more critical, epistemological perspective on the status of various statements about, for example, the perceived duration of mental events in heightened meditation (claimed to be on the order of milliseconds), or the clarity and stability of a mental image. Are these claims observational/phenomenological or theoretical? Are they spontaneous reports by yogi adepts, theoretical claims by philosopher scholars, or both? How do theory and observation relate in these sorts of statements?

We should also bear in mind the significant differences in the kinds of conversation possible between scientists and Western Buddhists and between scientists and Tibetan Buddhists, who have had little or no contact with Western culture or science. All four of the Western Buddhists at the ML XI meeting had experience in explaining the technical language of Buddhist philosophy to the uninitiated, and all deliberately edited their presentations in a way that would allow them to be maximally productive for the dialogue with scientists. In different ways, all focused on the empirical and rational aspects of Buddhism and minimized its more esoteric and explicitly spiritual dimensions.

In contrast, native Tibetan Buddhists with comparable monastic training have much greater difficulty in communicating to scientific audiences. They tend to speak simply out of the religious and esoteric, spiritual dimensions of their tradition, and in consequence scientists sometimes find themselves unable to make relevant connections. In this context, Princeton's Anne Triesman remarked, "I found Matthieu and Alan much more helpful than the Tibetans, not surprisingly, since they are aware of our background assumptions and know how to frame their explanations for our benefit." In constructing future collaborations it will be essential to bear these factors in mind.

With the help of funding from the Mind and Life Institute, several research collaborations are already under way that share the Davidson-Lutz-Ricard team's commitment to a genuinely collaborative sensibility. Each project faces its own unique methodological, theoretical, and practical challenges. For example, following a Mind and Life meeting in 2000, psychologist Paul Ekman and health psychologist Margaret Kemeny, both of the University of California, San Francisco, joined with Buddhist scholar-practitioner Alan Wallace to initiate a longitudinal study in which female teachers are trained in Buddhist methods intended to control destructive emotions and support emotional balance. The subjects are evaluated at three points in the study and compared with a control group. Stephen Kosslyn of Harvard has begun to evaluate the ability of meditators to generate and maintain mental imagery, and in a separate effort Jonathan Cohen of Princeton has initiated research into the capacity of meditators with respect to attention. In both of these areas, the exceptional claims made by Buddhist scholar-practitioners begged to be tested, and Kosslyn and Cohen independently rose to the challenge. Mind and Life has also made grants to psychologists Dacher Keltner at UC Berkeley and Daniel Reisberg at Reed College in related areas of study. Finally, the Santa Barbara Institute, headed by Alan Wallace, is pursuing two projects, a study with UC Davis on *shamatha* (mental quiescence), and one with UCLA on using meditation as an intervention for attention-deficit hyperactivity disorder.[4]

To foster the interest of young scientists in such research, in 2004 the Mind and Life Institute awarded small grants of up to $10,000 to ten investigators, all of whom attended the Mind and Life Summer Research Institute in 2004 (see below). These young investigators were eager to pursue a variety of questions raised in the course of the ML XI meeting, and to do so using a range of meditative approaches, from mindfulness-based stress reduction, as pioneered by Jon Kabat-Zinn, to Zen to Tibetan practices. While I cannot summarize all the projects, I will briefly describe two of them to offer a sense of the seriousness and sophistication of the efforts.

A graduate student at the Helen Willis Neuroscience Institute at UC Berkeley proposed to study *shamatha*, or sustained, undistracted, voluntary attention. More specifically, he proposed—based on prior evidence from the literature—that the amplitude of the steady-state somatosensory evoked potential (SSSEP) may be suitable as a real-time vigilance index, and in this sense function as a suitable neurophysiological correlate, or marker, for *shamatha*. He will evaluate the suitability of using this marker for an unusual population of patients who are about to receive subdural electrocorticographic electrode-grid implants to help manage intractable epilepsy. The implanted electrode grid may also provide a way to monitor the neural correlates of *shamatha*. Prior to implantation, the study group will receive training in mindfulness-based stress reduction; SSSEP will be used as a continuous measure of attention.

During the ML XI meeting, discussion took place concerning a level of human awareness termed metaconsciousness. Buddhist practitioners recognize this special mode of awareness and use it during meditation as the faculty that notices when, for example, attention has wandered from its meditative object. In a second research project, a graduate student at the Swartz Center for Computational Neuroscience at UC San Diego will study metacognition in both experienced Zen practitioners and naive subjects. While engaged in a meditative breathing practice, subjects will mark their metaconscious awareness of their mind's wandering by pushing a button. A 256-channel electroencephalogram (EEG) record will be analyzed prior to and following each button push to search for changes in the spectral and temporal neural dynamics, with special attention to the theta sources in the frontal midline area.

Using their small grants, other young researchers will investigate: attentional modulation in the visual cortex during meditation, executive function in attentional and emotional control, the functional plasticity of attention using advanced Zen meditators, and the neural and psychological mechanisms of therapeutic change associated with mindfulness meditation for social anxiety disorder. Concerning these grants, Richard Davidson wrote, "The fact that we've been able to provide ten seed grants to talented young scientists is wonderful and will ensure that research in this nascent area continues to flourish."

The Mind and Life Summer Research Institute

During the summer of 2004, and again in 2005, the Mind and Life Institute held a one-week summer research institute that aimed to follow up on a number of the questions and themes raised at the MIT meeting and provide an opportunity to explore empirical avenues for pursuing them further. The sessions were modeled to some degree on the well-known Cold Spring Harbor summer courses on molecular biology that were started by Max Delbrück and Salvador Luria in the 1940s. Delbrück and Luria's efforts are sometimes credited with educating a generation of biologists in the new quantitative and molecular methods that have become commonplace today. In the announcement of the 2004 Mind and Life Summer Research Institute (MLSRI), its goal was described as follows:[5]

The purpose of the Mind and Life Summer Research Institute is to advance collaborative research among cognitive and affective neuroscientists and Buddhist contemplative practitioners and scholars. The long-term objective is to advance the training of a new generation of cognitive/affective neuroscientists interested in exploring the influence of contemplative practice on mind, behavior, and brain function, including the potential role of contemplative methods for characterizing human experience and consciousness, and Buddhist scholars interested in expanding their knowledge of the modern mind sciences.

Fifty-nine graduate and postdoctoral students were admitted as research fellows, and thirty faculty members participated in the 2004 MLSRI as senior scholars. After the meeting, Richard Davidson wrote:

I found it to be an extraordinary event, both for how it was structured and for the topics it covered. The young scholars who were selected to participate were for the most part a very talented group. They came from the best universities in the country and were being trained very rigorously. A significant minority of the participants had an ongoing meditation practice, and they were longing for the kind of integration that we were providing. And to have it structured with significant amounts of meditation practice bracketing the scientific discussions was unlike any other scientific meeting I've ever attended. I believe it touched the participants very deeply and know that virtually all of the participants hope that it becomes a yearly fixture of M&L.

As Davidson observed, at least some and perhaps many of the participants were attempting to integrate two parts of their lives. Traditionally these two arenas of a person's life have been kept apart.

Within the science community there is an implicit and understandable code that urges us not to mingle personal religious commitments and scientific inquiry. The dangers of doing so are numerous and obvious. Creationist science is the classic example, where a pseudo-scientific account of evolution is produced to accommodate a particular interpretation of the biblical account of creation. Nonreligious ideologies can also distort science, as seen when practiced under both Nazi and Marxist regimes. If science is to benefit from its engagement with Buddhism, we should be clear about what if anything distinguishes Buddhism (or any comparable spiritual discipline or philosophy) from those dark instances where a divide is crossed with disastrous results. Noting this fact leads us to another major line of discussion that pervaded the MIT meeting, namely the relationship between knowledge and values.

Knowledge and Values

On the evening prior to the "Investigating the Mind" conference, the Department of Brain and Cognitive Sciences at MIT held an unusual meeting on Buddhist philosophy. Rajesh Kasturirangan, a student in the department completing his doctorate in theoretical cognitive science, was one of its participants. He described the room as filled with about fifty students and faculty—a substantial fraction of his department. People felt that something special was about to happen the next day, when the Dalai Lama would meet with cognitive scientists on MIT's campus. Later Kasturirangan wrote:

For me, the most memorable aspect of the Mind and Life conference held at MIT was not the conference itself, but the meeting we had in my department the night before the conference began. The meeting started out in a semi-academic manner, with a discussion of certain philosophical features of Buddhism. Then one of the persons in the room started talking about a personal tragedy and his inability to understand it, despite his professional training as a neuroscientist. While many people were made uneasy, I think it became clear that for many of the scientists in the room, their interest in Buddhism came from an unstated and perhaps uncomfortable disconnect between the models of cognitive science and neuroscience and their own experience as human beings. The possibility that Buddhism may offer a method that is as insightful about the subjective as science is about the objective intrigues many scientists. Whether the conference succeeded in legitimizing Buddhism as a worthy partner of cognitive/neuroscience is another question. What I will remember for a long time is the shared sense of having participated in something groundbreaking in that seminar room at MIT.

A related theme was developed by Harvard psychologist Jerome Kagan at the close of ML XI, when he reflected on what had led to such high interest in the ML XI meeting that it was heavily oversubscribed. Kagan drew attention to a fundamental difference in the attitudes of Buddhists and those in Western society toward the proper relationship between knowledge and values. We commonly portray the scientist as appropriately amoral, making her discoveries confident in the knowledge that knowing and ethics are disjunctive domains. This perceived divide runs deep in the Western tradition and has been generally accepted ever since David Hume distinguished between descriptive and prescriptive statements, between what "is" and what we "ought" to do. In theology, men such as Karl Barth reinforced the divide by advocating a neo-orthodox division of responsibility that granted the domain of natural knowledge to science while retaining moral judgment for religion. This division of territory has become so commonplace as to be nearly axiomatic for us, and yet the Buddhist scholar-practitioners at the ML XI meeting repeatedly argued for the credibility of an opposing view. In Buddhist philosophy, values and knowledge are inseparable. Because this runs counter to our own biases, it is worth rehearsing the arguments given in defense of this view.

The first is philosophical in character. Georges Dreyfus pointed out that as soon as the first-person perspective is included in one's method for the investigation of consciousness, interpretation is inevitably and intrinsically present. When we turn our attention to the outer world, we experience intentional objects. That is to say, our conscious awareness is always "about" something. Exactly what our awareness is about requires interpretation. Therefore, use of first-person experience necessarily entails interpretation, which in turn entails normative judgments. In this way ethics, either consciously or unconsciously, becomes part of cognition. Cognitive scientist Jonathan Cohen suggested that the "separation of church and state is a luxury tied to the fact that science has for so long primarily focused on the external and not the internal. If we take a pragmatist's view of ethics, as described here, and we say that ethics concerns internal states and suffering, and we now extend science to the study of those internal states through psychology and neuroscience, it may be that science no longer has the luxury of remaining separate from ethics."

The second argument takes its starting point from a Buddhist understanding of the goals of education in both its scholarly and its contemplative dimensions. Mastery of authoritative texts and logical reasoning are highly valued within Tibetan Buddhist monastic education, as they are in Western higher education. Such mastery, however, is complemented by a vigorous contemplative pedagogy whose objective is not merely the mastery of philosophical or religious knowledge but the transformation of the individual. As emphasized repeatedly by the Buddhists, the mind is, in their view, malleable, and the purpose of meditation is its transformation, for example to overcome the three mental toxins of hatred, craving, and mental delusion. Meditation is the primary means for transforming the aspirant to a new way of living and experiencing that leads to liberation, which is understood as freedom from affliction. In this view, who we "become" is of paramount significance in human development, not only what we know. Academic erudition is an essential component of education, but according to Buddhist thinking, the false views of world and self that cause suffering must not only be understood abstractly but also lived. An education of this type is inherently ethical. Although there are vocal advocates in the West for transformative learning, such as Jack Mezirow of Columbia and Robert Kegan at Harvard, it has played a relatively minor role in Western ideas of education. Instead the emphasis has been on critical reasoning, the mastery of a body of established knowledge, and the acquisition of marketable skills.

During the dialogue on emotions at the MIT meeting, Berkeley psychology professor Dacher Keltner contrasted the scientific view of emotions as short-lived transient effects with the long process of establishing enduring emotions as they are understood in Buddhism. In the same session, the Dalai Lama contrasted emotional outbursts with more enduring emotions, such as compassion, which are the hard-won fruits of reason and meditation. He said, "Other types of emotions can be seen as reason-based, where as a result of a long process of contemplation, such as cultivating compassion, you arrive at a point of very strong feeling, such as the intense feeling of compassion. That kind of emotion is grounded in a more reasoned reflection. I feel that a distinction needs to be made between these two types of emotion."

Buddhist education is focused on identifying the negative or destructive factors that lead to obscuration and thus to suffering, and on devising pedagogical strategies (meditation among them) that can counter these negative factors in the human personality and so promote insight. The Buddhist goal of enlightenment is simultaneously a knowledge project and an ethical project.

The third argument offered by the Buddhist perspective for questioning the knowledge-value divide comes out of the Buddhist understanding of ethics. As Jerome Kagan pointed out, in the Western view, whether a scientist is a good or bad person with altruistic or selfish motives is seen as irrelevant to the science itself. Science is value neutral. In Buddhist ethics the division is not so tidy. This difference came to the fore during the 2002 Mind and Life dialogue in Dharamsala, when Eric Lander and the Dalai Lama wrestled with the difficult ethical issues raised by genetic engineering. One consideration brought forward by the Dalai Lama surprised Lander. In Buddhist ethical reasoning, motivation is an essential factor in determining whether an action is ethically proper or improper. The identical action can be ethically positive or negative, depending on the motivation. For example, if greed is the motive for a scientific research project, this might be enough to convert an otherwise ethically positive activity into one that is negative.

In his closing remarks at MIT, Kagan declared that humans are uniquely "ethical animals." Unlike all other animals, we judge our experiences as good or bad. In addition Kagan reminded us that, since the Enlightenment, the noble view of human nature has increasingly come under attack by social forces as well as by the declarations of modern science. As a result, he said, "None of us should be surprised that many Americans became eager for any scientific evidence or philosophical argument that could challenge this dark, materialistic view of human nature." As he put it, "Humans do not like to think of themselves as jackals." If Western society and science depict us in this manner, then we will seek alternatives. Human concerns may not be divided so neatly between knowledge and values, or science and religion. People will seek worldviews that allow them to undertake science with rigor and passion, and also to preserve a high-minded and dignified view of our humanity. The enormous public interest in the ML XI meeting supported Kagan's judgment that any serious attempt to reconcile the sciences with those spiritual traditions that affirm humanity's high nature would be most welcome.

Conclusion

Speaking personally, I believe that the cognitive science students at MIT were right in feeling that something historic might be afoot. For the two days spent "investigating the mind" at MIT, two great traditions came together before a large audience of scholars and scientists. More than a hundred media representatives were present as well, and a flood of reports were published in scientific journals and the mainstream media. While the meeting itself was only the beginning of a conversation and collaboration, we should remember that it was the fruit of sixteen years of Mind and Life dialogues between scientists and the Dalai Lama. These dialogues, together with the new summer research institutes, grants, and collaborative projects, all need to continue if the seeds planted at MIT are to grow and flourish in the coming decades. However, Buddhism need not be the only partner in this enterprise. It merely exemplifies a form of what the Dalai Lama calls secular spirituality—that is to say, a spirituality that is simultaneously committed to experience (including meditative experience) and reason, while being embedded in what he terms "secular ethics." I am not a Buddhist, but I do share the Dalai Lama's conviction that science can be conjoined to a high ethical and spiritual understanding of the human being. I am one of those, described by Kagan, who rejects the "dark, materialistic view of human nature." I see no reason why science cannot move boldly to extend its domain of exploration to include the human mind without diminishing the human being in the slightest.

I would like to conclude by recalling the words of Charles Vest, president of MIT, when he opened the conference: "There is no more profound or worthy subject of study than how we learn, remember, think, and communicate—in other words, how the brain works and what the mind is." In the meeting recorded in this volume, we took several modest steps toward "the ultimate mystery of consciousness." It required us to reach beyond normal interdisciplinary dialogue because, in the words of Vest, "At the most profound level these studies challenge those of us in the sciences and technologies to go still further afield, to grapple with insights and challenges from the world's great philosophical and spiritual traditions." As we travel ever farther afield, we are engaged not in a flight from science but rather in a worthy extension of its methods and domains.

ABOUT THE MIND AND LIFE INSTITUTE
CONTRIBUTORS
NOTES
INDEX

R. ADAM ENGLE

About the Mind and Life Institute

The Mission of the Mind and Life Institute

The Mind and Life Institute is grounded in a commitment to dialogue between Western science and the Eastern contemplative traditions, especially Buddhism. Its goal is to discover how the persistent and courageous mutual interrogation of different knowledge traditions might help advance our understanding of the nature of reality—especially of the human mind—and to explore how such understanding may be used to promote well-being on the planet. Over the eighteen years of its existence, the Mind and Life Institute has had a privileged partnership with the Dalai Lama of Tibet, and the Mind and Life dialogues with the Dalai Lama have covered topics ranging from physics and cosmology to neuroplasticity, from altruism and ethics to destructive emotions.

The work of the Mind and Life Institute begins with dialogue, but it does not end there. We are also committed to finding strategies for translating new understandings into programs, interventions, and tools that will bring tangible benefit to people's lives. To this end we have recently, as an organization, begun to ask our dialogue process to explore a series of very practical questions. How do we create and maintain a healthy mind and brain? How can we cultivate more emotional balance in our lives and our society? How can we teach self-management skills conducive to emotional balance earlier in life?

Mind and Life currently operates through four divisions, all working synergistically in the service of its two-pronged mission of understanding and service:

1. *Mind and Life Dialogues* set the scientific agenda by exploring which areas of science are most ripe for collaboration and how collaboration can be implemented most effectively.
2. *Mind and Life Publications* report to the greater scientific community and the interested public on what has occurred at our dialogue sessions.
3. *The Mind and Life Summer Research Institute* is an annual weeklong residential symposium, targeted for younger researchers and practitioners in particular, that aims to train a new generation for the complex tasks of pursuing rigorous collaborative work at the interface of science (especially biobehavioral and biomedical science) and contemplative practice.
4. *The Mind and Life Research Grant Program* provides seed grants to investigate hypotheses formulated at or explored during the Mind and Life dialogues and at the research institute.

A History of the Mind and Life Institute

The Mind and Life dialogues between His Holiness the Dalai Lama and Western scientists were brought to life through a collaboration between myself, R. Adam Engle, a North American businessman, and Francisco J. Varela, a Chilean-born neuroscientist living and working in Paris. In 1984, before we had met, Varela and I each independently developed proposals to create a series of cross-cultural meetings at which the Dalai Lama and scientists from the West would engage in extended discussion over a period of days.

In deciding to partner on this effort, we adopted several operating principles that proved to be critical to the subsequent success of the Mind and Life series. Perhaps the most important was that scientists would not be chosen solely by their reputation, or by their competence in their domain, but also by their open-mindedness. Some familiarity with Buddhism was helpful but not essential. What was key, we decided, was a healthy respect for the dialogue and an openness to the potential insights to be gained from representatives from Eastern contemplative traditions.

To ensure that the meetings would be fully participatory, they were structured with presentations by Western scientists in the morning session, allowing His Holiness to be briefed on the basic ground of a field of knowledge. Each morning presentation was based on a broad, mainstream, and balanced scientific point of view. Each afternoon session was devoted solely to discussion of questions and issues that naturally flowed from the morning presentation. During these discussion sessions, the morning presenter was free to state his or her personal preferences and judgments, even if they differed from more generally accepted viewpoints.

The curriculum for the first Mind and Life dialogue (Mind and Life I) introduced various broad themes from cognitive science, touching on scientific method, neurobiology, cognitive psychology, artificial intelligence, brain development, and evolution; Francisco Varela was the scientific coordinator. The event, which was held in Dharamsala, India, was an enormously gratifying success: both His Holiness and the participants felt that there was a true meeting of minds, and that some substantial advances were made in bridging the gap between Western science and Eastern Buddhism. At the conclusion of the meeting, the Dalai Lama encouraged us to continue with further dialogues.

Mind and Life I was transcribed, edited, and published as *Gen-*

tle Bridges: Conversations with the Dalai Lama on the Sciences of Mind, edited by Jeremy W. Hayward and Francisco J. Varela (Boston: Shambhala Publications, 1992). This book has been translated into French, Spanish, German, Japanese, and Chinese.

Mind and Life II took place in October 1989 in Newport, California. The emphasis of this two-day event was on brain sciences, specifically neuroscience, and Robert Livingston was the scientific coordinator. The event was especially memorable because His Holiness was awarded the Nobel Peace Prize on the first morning of the meeting. The proceedings of this meeting are reported in *Consciousness at the Crossroads: Conversations with the Dalai Lama on Brain Science and Buddhism*, edited by Zara Houshmand, Robert B. Livingstone, and B. Allan Wallace (Boston: Snow Lion Publications, 1999).

Mind and Life III returned to Dharamsala in 1990. Daniel Goleman served as scientific coordinator for the meeting, which focused on the relationship between emotions and health. The volume covering Mind and Life III is *Healing Emotions: Conversations with the Dalai Lama on Mindfulness, Emotions, and Health*, edited by Daniel Goleman (Boston: Shambhala Publications, 1997).

The fourth Mind and Life conference took place in October 1992, with Francisco Varela again acting as scientific coordinator. The topic for the dialogue was sleep, dreams, and dying. The account of this conference can be found in the volume *Sleeping, Dreaming, and Dying: An Exploration of Consciousness with the Dalai Lama*, edited by Francisco J. Varela (Boston: Wisdom Publications, 1997).

Mind and Life V was also held in Dharamsala, in April 1995. The topic was altruism, ethics, and compassion, and the scientific coordinator was Richard Davidson. The volume covering this meeting is *Visions of Compassion: Western Scientists and Tibetan Buddhists Examine Human Nature*, edited by Richard J. Davidson and Anne Harrington (New York: Oxford University Press, 2002).

Mind and Life VI opened a new area of exploration beyond the life sciences. The meeting, which focused on physics, took place in Dharamsala in October 1997, with Arthur Zajonc as the scientific coordinator. The resulting volume is *The New Physics and Cosmology*, edited by Arthur Zajonc (Oxford: Oxford University Press, 2003). The dialogue on quantum physics was continued with Mind and Life VII, held in June 1998 at the Institute for Experimental Physics, directed by Anton Zeilinger, in Innsbruck, Austria. That meeting was written up in the January 1999 issue of Germany's *Geo* magazine.

Mind and Life VIII was held in March 2000 in Dharamsala, with Daniel Goleman acting again as scientific coordinator. The subject of this meeting was destructive emotions. The volume reporting on this meeting is *Destructive Emotions: How Can We Overcome Them? A Scientific Dialogue with the Dalai Lama*, edited by Daniel Goleman (New York: Bantam, 2003). This book has been translated into more than thirty languages.

Mind and Life IX was held in 2001 at the University of Wisconsin–Madison in cooperation with the HealthEmotions Research Institute and the Center for Research on Mind-Body Interactions. The meeting focused on how to most effectively use the technologies of functional magnetic resonance imaging (fMRI) and electroencephalography/magnetoencephalography (EEG/MEG) in research on meditation, perception, and emotion, and on the relations between human neural plasticity and meditation practices.

Mind and Life X was held in Dharamsala in October 2002. The topic was "What Is Matter? What Is Life?" and Arthur Zajonc acted as scientific coordinator and moderator. The editors of the volume about this meeting are Luigi Luisi and Zara Houshmand.

Mind and Life XI, "Investigating the Mind: Exchanges between Buddhism and the Biobehavioral Sciences on How the Mind Works," the subject of this book, was the first public meeting in the Mind and Life series. It took place on the campus of the Massachusetts Institute of Technology in Cambridge, Massachusetts, on September 13 and 14, 2003, and was cosponsored by the McGovern Institute at MIT.

Mind and Life XII was held in Dharamsala in October 2004. The subject of the meeting was neuroplasticity, and the scientific coordinator was Richard Davidson. The forthcoming book about this meeting, written by Sharon Begley, will be published by Random House in early 2007.

Mind and Life XIII, "The Science and Clinical Applications of Meditation," was held in Washington, D.C., in November 2005 and was cohosted by the Georgetown Medical Center and Johns Hopkins Medical School. The scientific coordinators were Richard Davidson and Jon Kabat-Zinn.

The Mind and Life Institute began a laboratory research program in 2000 to test some of the hypotheses developed in its meetings. As of this writing, Mind and Life has awarded grants to twenty-six investigators in the fields of psychology and neuroscience. Articles reporting the results of these studies have begun to appear in such journals as the *Proceedings of the National Academy of Sciences*. In 2004 Mind and Life launched the Mind and Life Summer Research Institute, an annual, week-long residential symposium for graduate students, postdoctoral students, and senior investigators, to further advance efforts at research collaboration between scientists and contemplatives.

The Mind and Life Institute headquarters are in Louisville, Colorado. More information may be found on the Web site www.mindandlife.org.

Contributors

AJAHN AMARO is currently co-abbot of Abhayagiri Buddhist Monastery in northern California. He is the author of three books—*Tudong: The Long Road North, Silent Rain,* and *Small Boat, Great Mountain: Theravadan Reflections on the Natural Great Perfection*—and the editor of *The Pilgrim Kamanita.* A new book, *The Island: An Anthology of the Buddha's Teachings on Nirvana,* is forthcoming. After receiving a degree in psychology and physiology from London University, in 1977 Amaro took up residence in a forest meditation monastery in the lineage of Venerable Ajahn Chah in Northeast Thailand. He went on to serve in positions of leadership in forest monasteries in England for many years. The Abhayagiri Monastery opened in 1996.

MARLENE BEHRMANN is professor of psychology at Carnegie Mellon University and has appointments at the Center for the Neural Basis of Cognition (Carnegie Mellon University and University of Pittsburgh) and in the departments of neuroscience and communication disorders at the University of Pittsburgh. Her many honors include the American Psychological Association Distinguished Scientific Award for Early Career Contributions to Behavioral and Cognitive Neuroscience, the Presidential Early Career Award in Science and Engineering, and the American Psychological Early Career Award in Neuropsychology.

JONATHAN COHEN is professor of psychology, director of the Center for the Study of Brain, Mind, and Behavior, and director of the Program in Neuroscience at Princeton University. He is also associate professor of psychiatry at the University of Pittsburgh School of Medicine. He has received the National Institute of Mental Health (NIMH) Training Award in Psychiatry; the Annual Resident Research Award, Northern California Psychiatric Society; the Miller Foundation Prize for Research in Psychiatry and Behavioral Sciences; the NIMH Physician Scientist Award; the NIMH First Award; the Joseph Zubin Memorial Fund Award for Research in Psychopathology; and the Kempf Fund Award.

RICHARD J. DAVIDSON is the William James and Vilas Research Professor of Psychology and Psychiatry and director of the W. M. Keck Laboratory for Functional Brain Imaging and Behavior at the University of Wisconsin–Madison. He is internationally recognized for his research on the neural substrates of emotion and emotional disorders, and has published more than 150 articles on these topics. He has also contributed many chapters and reviews, and has edited nine books. His many awards include a National Institute of Mental Health Research Scientist Award, a Merit Award from NIMH, an Established Investigator Award from the National Alliance for Research in Schizophrenia and Affective Disorders, the William James Fellow Award from the American Psychological Society, and the Hilldale Award from the University of Wisconsin–Madison.

GEORGES DREYFUS is professor of religion and chair of the Department of Religion at Williams College. His languages of specialization include Tibetan, Sanskrit, and Pali. He serves as cochair for the Tibetan and Himalayan Religions Group at the American Academy of Religion and is also a member of the Academy Steering Committee. He has published five books, including *Tibetan Interpretations* and *The Sound of Two Hands Clapping: The Education of a Tibetan Buddhist Monk*, along with many articles. His awards include a Foreign Language Area Study Fellowship in 1988–89, a Fulbright Fellowship to India in 1989–90, and a National Endowment for the Humanities award in 1994–95.

R. ADAM ENGLE is the cofounder and chairman of the Mind and Life Institute. He holds a law degree and a masters in business administration from Harvard and Stanford, respectively. He first came into contact with the Tibetan community in 1974 and has been working for Tibetan causes since then. In addition to running the Mind and Life Institute, he is the founder of the Colorado Friends of Tibet, a statewide Tibetan support group based in Boulder, and he previously established a speaker's series at the Stanford Business School entitled "Integrity and Compassion in Business." His other affiliations include founding membership in the Social Venture Network and membership in the World Business Academy.

DANIEL GILBERT is professor of psychology at Harvard University. He has won the American Psychological Association's Distinguished Scientific Award for an Early Career Contribution to Psychology, has received fellowships from the John Simon Guggenheim Memorial Foundation and the American Philosophical Society, and has been a fellow at Stanford University's Center for Advanced Research in the Behavioral Sciences. His numerous chapters and research articles in psychology are concerned especially with his work on affective forecasting. He is also the author of several works of science fiction and the editor of *The Handbook of Social Psychology*.

TENZIN GYATSO is the Fourteenth Dalai Lama, the leader of Tibetan Buddhism, the head of the Tibetan government-in-exile, and a spiritual leader revered worldwide. The Dalai Lamas are believed by Buddhists to be manifestations of the Buddha of Compassion, who chooses to reincarnate for the purpose of serving human beings. Winner of the Nobel Peace Prize in 1989, the Dalai Lama is universally respected as a spokesman for the compassionate and peaceful resolution of human conflict. He is the author of many books published in English, the most recent being a series of reflections on his lifelong engagement with modern science.

ANNE HARRINGTON is Loeb Harvard College Professor and professor for the history of science at Harvard University, specializing in the history of psychiatry, neuroscience, and the other mind sciences. She also holds a visiting professorship at the London School of Economics, where she is based at the BIOS Centre for Social Studies of the Life Sciences. For six years, she was codirector of the Harvard Interfaculty Mind/Brain/Behavior Initiative, an interdisciplinary venture at the interface of neuroscience, the humanities, and the social sciences. She also served as a consultant for the MacArthur Foundation Research Network on Mind-Body Interactions from 1993 through 1999. In addition to many articles and chapters, her books include *Medicine, Mind and the Double Brain; Reenchanted Science; The Placebo Effect* (editor); and *Stories under the Skin* (forthcoming).

THUPTEN JINPA is currently president and editor-in-chief of the Institute of Tibetan Classics, a nonprofit educational organization dedicated to translating key Tibetan classics into contemporary languages. He was educated in classical Tibetan monastic academia and received the highest academic degree of Geshe Lharam (equivalent to a doctorate in divinity). He also holds degrees in philosophy and religious studies from the University of Cambridge. Since 1985 he has been the principal English-language translator to the Dalai Lama. He has published a range of scholarly articles on Tibetan culture and

Buddhism. His two latest works are *Songs of Spiritual Experience: Tibetan Poems of Awakening and Insight* (coauthored with Jaś Elsner) and *Self, Reality and Reason in Tibetan Thought*.

JEROME KAGAN is Daniel and Amy Starch Research Professor of Psychology at Harvard University and a member of the Board on Neuroscience and Biobehavioral Research at the Institute of Medicine. The focus of his research for the past twenty years has been the relation between the infant temperamental qualities of high and low reactivity and the subsequent development of variations in mood and behavior that are called inhibited and uninhibited. He is a recipient of the Distinguished Scientist Award given by the American Psychological Association and the Distinguished Scientist Award given by the Society for Research in Child Development.

DANIEL KAHNEMAN is Eugene Higgins Professor of Psychology and professor of public affairs at the Woodrow Wilson School, Princeton University. His research interests include basic processes of vision, pupillary measures of effort, and the role of grouping factors in visual attention. In collaboration with Amos Tversky he has studied judgmental heuristics and framing effects in decision making. He has also done research on fairness in economic decision making, the valuation of public goods, and the psychology of juries. He is a recipient of the Distinguished Scientific Contribution Award of the American Psychological Association and the Hilgard Award for Career Contribution to General Psychology, and of an honorary doctorate from the University of Pennsylvania. He is a member of the American Academy of Arts and Sciences, the National Academy of Sciences, and the Econometric Society.

NANCY KANWISHER is a professor in the Department of Brain and Cognitive Sciences at MIT and an investigator at the McGovern Institute for Brain Research. Her research, which makes use of behavioral methods, functional magnetic resonance imaging, and magnetoencephalography, is concerned with the cognitive and neural mechanisms underlying visual experience, particularly visual object recognition. Kanwisher received a MacArthur Foundation Fellowship in Peace and International Security in 1986, a National Institute of Mental Health First Award in 1988, a Troland Research Award from the National Academy of Sciences in 1999, and a MacVicar Faculty Fellow Award from MIT in 2002.

DACHER KELTNER is professor of psychology at the University of California, Berkeley, and director of the Berkeley Center for the Development of Peace and Well-being. His awards include the 2001 Positive Psychology prize for research excellence, the 2002 Western Psychological Association prize for outstanding research for an investigator under forty, and a UC Berkeley Letters and Science Distinguished Teaching Award.

STEPHEN M. KOSSLYN is John Lindsley Professor of Psychology at Harvard University and associate psychologist in the Department of Neurology at Massachusetts General Hospital. His research has focused primarily on the nature of visual mental imagery, visual perception, and visual communication; he has published seven books and more than two hundred papers on these topics. He has received the American Psychological Association's Boyd R. McCandless Young Scientist Award, the National Academy of Sciences Initiatives in Research Award, the Cattell Award, the J.-L. Signoret Prize (France), and has been elected to Academia Rodinensis pro Remediatione (Switzerland), the American Academy of Arts and Sciences, and the Society of Experimental Psychologists.

ERIC LANDER is professor of biology at the Massachusetts Institute of Technology. He is a geneticist, a molecular biologist, a mathematician, a founding director of the Broad Institute, and one of the principal leaders of the Human Genome Project. From 1981 to 1990 he was assistant and then associate professor of managerial economics at the Harvard Business School. He was named a Rhodes Scholar in 1978, and he received a MacArthur Foundation Fellowship in 1987 for his work in genetics. In 1997, he was elected to the National Academy of Sciences; in 1998, to the Institute of Medicine; and in 1999, to the American Academy of Arts and Sciences.

DAVID E. MEYER is a mathematical psychologist and cognitive scientist on the faculty of the Cognition and Perception Program in the Department of Psychology at the University of Michigan, Ann Arbor. After receiving his doctorate, he worked for almost a decade as a member of the technical staff in the Human Information Processing Research Department at Bell Telephone Laboratories before returning to academic research and teaching. His many affiliations include elected fellowships in the Society of Experimental Psychologists, the American Psychological Society, the American Psychological Association, and the American Association for the Advancement of Science.

DANIEL REISBERG is professor of psychology at Reed College. In his research he has explored the conscious experience of imagery, and how this experience influences remembering and problem solving. His research interests also include how people remember the emotional events of their lives, and he is currently coeditor of a new book on this topic. He has published more than fifty chapters and journal articles, and he serves on the editorial boards of many research journals.

MATTHIEU RICARD has been a Buddhist monk for twenty years at Shechen Monastery in Nepal, and he is the French interpreter for the Dalai Lama. He holds a doctorate in cell genetics from the Institut Pasteur and is the author of the widely read book *Animal Migrations* (1969). In his capacity as a Tibetan Buddhist monk and scholar, he has also written *The Monk and the Philosopher*, a book of dialogues with his father, the French philosopher Jean-François Revel, and *The Quantum and the Lotus,* a dialogue with the astrophysicist Trinh Xuan Thuan. For his numerous contributions to society, he was awarded knighthood in the French National Order of Merit.

EVAN THOMPSON is associate professor of philosophy at York University, where he holds the Canada Research Chair in Cognitive Science and the Embodied Mind. His books include *The Embodied Mind: Cognitive Science and Human Experience* (written with Francisco Varela and Eleanor Rosch), *Colour Vision: A Study in Cognitive Science and the Philosophy of Perception, Between Ourselves: Second-Person Issues in the Study of Consciousness,* and *Vision and Mind: Selected Readings in the Philosophy of Perception* (written with Alva Noë). He is currently finishing a book, begun with the late Francisco Varela, titled *Radical Embodiment: The Lived Body in Biology, Cognitive Science, and Human Experience.* He is a member of the McDonnell Project in Philosophy and the Neurosciences, and in 2003 was a visiting senior scholar at the Centre de Recherche en Epistémologie Appliqué (CREA), at the Ecole Polytechnique in Paris.

ANNE TREISMAN is the James S. McDonnell Distinguished University Professor at Princeton University. She is a member of the Royal Society, London; the National Academy, USA; the American Academy of Arts and Sciences; and the Society of Experimental Psychologists; and is an elected fellow in the American Psychological Society. Her awards include a Killam Senior Fellowship, the James McKeen Cattell Sabbatical Award, the Howard Crosby Warren Medal of the Society of Experimental Psychologists, the Distinguished Scientific Contribution Award of the American Psychological Association, and the Golden Brain Award of the Minerva Foundation (for "fundamental breakthroughs that extend our knowledge of vision and the brain").

B. ALAN WALLACE is president of the Santa Barbara Institute for the Interdisciplinary Study of Consciousness. He trained for many years as a monk in Buddhist monasteries in India and Switzerland. He has taught Buddhist theory and practice in Europe and the United States since 1976 and has served as interpreter for numerous Tibetan scholars and contemplatives, including the Dalai Lama. He has edited, translated, authored, and contributed to more than thirty books on Tibetan Buddhism, medicine, language, and culture, and the interface more generally between science and religion. His published works include *Choosing Reality: A Buddhist View of Physics and the Mind* (1996), *The Bridge of Quiescence: Experiencing Buddhist Meditation* (1998), *The Taboo of Subjectivity: Toward a New Science of Consciousness* (2000), and *Buddhism and Science: Breaking New Ground* (2003).

ARTHUR ZAJONC is professor of physics at Amherst College, where he has taught since 1978. Over the years, he has been a visiting professor and research scientist at the Ecole Normale Superieure in Paris, the Max Planck Institute for Quantum Optics, the University of Rochester, and the universities of Hannover and Innsbruck in Austria. He is author of the book *Catching the Light*, coauthor of *The Quantum Challenge*, and coeditor of *Goethe's Way of Science*.

Notes

1. Introduction

1. For the standard introduction to the historical issues here, see David Lindberg and Ronald Numbers, eds., *God and Nature: Historical Essays on the Encounter between Christianity and Science* (Berkeley: University of California Press, 1986); also John Brooke and Geoffrey Cantor, *Reconstructing Nature: The Engagement of Science and Religion* (New York: Oxford University Press, 1998).

2. More particularly, in the "Prologemena" to his 1893 *Evolution and Ethics*, Huxley offered what was for the time a remarkably detailed and sympathetic analysis of Buddhism, writing in part:

> With just insight into human nature, Gautama declared extreme ascetic practices to be useless and indeed harmful. The appetites and the passions are not to be abolished by mere mortification of the body; they must, in addition, be attacked on their own ground and

conquered by steady cultivation of the mental habits which oppose them; by universal benevolence; by the return of good for evil; by humility; by abstinence from evil thought; in short, by total renunciation of that self-assertion which is the essence of the cosmic process.

Doubtless, it is to these ethical qualities that Buddhism owes its marvellous success. A system which knows no God in the western sense; which denies a soul to man; which counts the belief in immortality a blunder and the hope of it a sin; which refuses any efficacy to prayer and sacrifice; which bids men look to nothing but their own efforts for salvation; which, in its original purity, knew nothing of vows of obedience, abhorred intolerance, and never sought the aid of the secular arm; yet spread over a considerable moiety of the Old World with marvellous rapidity, and is still, with whatever base admixture of foreign superstitions, the dominant creed of a large fraction of mankind.

For a further discussion of the place of Buddhism in Huxley's projects, see Vijitha Rajapakse, "Buddhism in Huxley's Evolution and Ethics: A Note on a Victorian Evaluation and Its 'Comparativist Dimension,'" *Philosophy East and West* 35, no. 3 (July 1985): 295–304.

3. Agehananda Bharati, "The Hindu Renaissance and Its Apologetic Patterns," *Journal of Asian Studies* 29 (Feb. 1970): 267–287.

4. For a good overview of this tradition, see Franz Aubrey Metcalf, "The Encounter of Buddhism and Psychology," in *Westward Dharma: Buddhism beyond Asia*, ed. Charles S. Prebish and Martin Baumann (Berkeley: University of California Press, 2002), 348–363.

5. See such Mind and Life Institute publications as *Healing Emotions: Conversations with the Dalai Lama on Mindfulness, Emotions, and Health*, ed. Daniel Goleman (Boston: Shambhala, 1997), and *Destructive Emotions: How Can We Overcome Them? A Scientific Dialogue with the Dalai Lama*, ed. Daniel Goleman (New York: Bantam, 2003).

6. Humberto R. Maturana and Francisco J. Varela, *Autopoiesis and Cognition: The Realization of the Living* (Boston: D. Reidel, 1980).

7. Francisco J. Varela, "The Importance of the Encounter with Buddhism for Modern Science," online at the Mind and Life Institute Web site, www.mindandlife.com/encounter.html.

8. Donald S. Lopez, Jr., "New Age Orientalism: The Case of Tibet,"

Tricycle: The Buddhist Review 3, no. 3 (1994): 38. Orientalism is a term invented in 1970 by the Palestinian literary scholar Edward Said, who stressed the ways in which these habits of thinking have historically functioned to sanction the varied imperialist and interventionist ambitions of the Western colonialist powers. Thus, for example, the writings of nineteenth-century Christian missionaries, colonial administrators, and passing travelers were filled with descriptions of the Orient or the East as an exotic place filled with primitive despots, self-flagellating penitents, yogis who lived lives wholly detached from the world, and indolent opium eaters. Typically, these descriptions were then contrasted with the civilized, rational, modern, and pragmatic world of their authors. What Lopez and others are talking about is an inversion in our own time of the original moral logic of orientalism: the West is now the deficient party that needs to be put right by Eastern understandings and practices.

9. Ricard's work was carried out in collaboration with Richard Davidson of the University of Wisconsin at Madison. In an interview done just before the MIT conference for the Australian radio program *All in the Mind*, Ricard spoke of the compatibility between his Buddhist practices and his new work with Davidson: "I was investigating genetics and mapping the chromosome of some bacteria and then for me it was just a straight line to continue in what I call 'contemplative science,' because science is about discovery, but here the domain is the mind looking at itself. We always imagine science with a lot of complicated apparatus, but if it is the mind trying to investigate itself—by looking at how the thoughts arise, how the emotions form, how they multiply, how they invade your mind, how you could possibly disengage your mind from being a slave of those emotions—so in that you have the best apparatus since you are born and until you die." "Meditation and the Mind: Science Meets Buddhism," *All in the Mind: With Natasha Mitchell*, Sept. 14, 2003, www.abc.net.au/rn/science/mind/s943369.htm.

10. Gareth Cook, "Dalai Lama Visit Provides a Subject for Scientists," *Boston Globe*, Sept. 12, 2003, www.boston.com/news/nation/articles/2003/09/12/dalai_lama_visit_provides_a_subject_for_scientists.

11. "Genome Center Director Eric Lander to Visit His Holiness the Dalai Lama," *Whitehead Institute for Biomedical Research*, Sept. 30, 2002, www.wi.mit.edu/news/archives/2002/el_0930.html; "Mind and

Life X: The Nature of Matter, the Nature of Life," *Mind and Life Institute*, www.mindandlife.com/conf02.html.

12. Swati Chopra, "Buddhism's Dialogue with Science," *Times News Network*, Oct. 6, 2002, www.purifymind.com/DialogueScience .htm.

13. Robert Reinhold, "Exiled Lama Teaches Americans Buddhist Tenets Periled in Tibet," *New York Times*, July 24, 1973, 22.

14. Jeffery Paine, "The Buddha of Suburbia: The Dalai Lama's American Religion," *Boston Globe*, Sept. 14, 2003, www.boston.com/ news/globe/ideas/articles/2003/09/14/the_buddha_of_suburbia.

15. For more on Thurman's larger cultural and advocacy roles, see Rodger Kamenetz, "Robert Thurman Doesn't Look Buddhist," *New York Times Magazine*, May 5, 1996, 46–49.

16. For more on the use of Shangri-la imagery in contemporary discussions of Tibet, both popular and scholarly, see the controversial work of Donald S. Lopez, Jr., *Prisoners of Shangri-La: Tibetan Buddhism and the West* (Chicago: University of Chicago Press, 1998). For a discussion of earlier Western constructions of Tibet as a uniquely sacred, pristine world, see Peter Bishop, *The Myth of Shangri-La: Tibet, Travel Writing, and the Western Creation of a Sacred Landscape* (Berkeley: University of California Press, 1989).

17. Thupten Jinpa, "Science as an Ally or a Rival Philosophy? Tibetan Buddhist Thinkers' Engagement with Modern Science," in *Buddhism and Science: Breaking New Ground*, ed. B. Alan Wallace (New York: Columbia University Press, 2003).

18. Goleman, ed., *Destructive Emotions*.

19. These comments were conveyed to Thupten Jinpa by the Dalai Lama in private conversation. See Jinpa, "Science as an Ally?"

2. Neurophenomenology and Francisco Varela

1. Representative examples of his contributions to these fields include, in neuroscience, Francisco J. Varela et al., "The Brainweb: Phase Synchronization and Large-Scale Integration," *Nature Reviews Neuroscience* 2 (2001): 229–239; in immunology, Francisco J. Varela and Antonio Coutinho, "Second-Generation Immune Networks," *Immunology Today* 12 (1991): 159–166; in theoretical biology, Francisco J. Varela,

Principles of Biological Autonomy (New York: North Holland, 1979); in cognitive science, Francisco J. Varela, Evan Thompson, and Eleanor Rosch, *The Embodied Mind: Cognitive Science and Human Experience* (Cambridge, MA: MIT Press, 1991). On the exchange between Buddhism and science, see Varela, Thompson, and Rosch, *Embodied Mind;* Jeremy W. Hayward and Francisco J. Varela, eds., *Gentle Bridges: Conversations with the Dalai Lama on the Sciences of Mind* (Boston: Shambhala, 1992); Francisco J. Varela, ed., *Sleeping, Dreaming, and Dying: An Exploration of Consciousness with the Dalai Lama* (Boston: Wisdom, 1997); Francisco J. Varela and Nathalie Depraz, "Imagination: Embodiment, Phenomenology, and Transformation," in *Buddhism and Science: Breaking New Ground*, ed. B. Alan Wallace (New York: Columbia University Press, 2003), 195–232.

2. Eugenio Rodriguez et al., "Perception's Shadow: Long-Distance Synchronization of Human Brain Activity," *Nature* 397 (1999): 430–433; Michel Le Van Quyen et al., "Anticipation of Epileptic Seizures from Standard EEG Recordings," *Lancet* 357 (2001): 183–188; Varela, "The Brainweb"; Evan Thompson and Francisco J. Varela, "Radical Embodiment: Neural Dynamics and Consciousness," *Trends in Cognitive Sciences* 5 (2001): 418–425; Antoine Lutz et al., "Guiding the Study of Brain Dynamics by Using First-Person Data: Synchrony Patterns Correlate with Ongoing Conscious States during a Simple Visual Task," *Proceedings of the National Academy of Sciences USA* 99 (2002): 1586–1591.

3. William James, *The Principles of Psychology* (Cambridge, MA: Harvard University Press, 1981), 185.

4. Ibid.

5. Ibid., 236–237.

6. See Eugene Taylor, *William James on Consciousness beyond the Margin* (Princeton: Princeton University Press, 1996), 147.

7. James McKeen Cattell, "The Conceptions and Methods of Psychology," *Popular Science Monthly* 60 (1904), as quoted in William Lyons, *The Disappearance of Introspection* (Cambridge, MA: MIT Press, 1986), 23.

8. B. Alan Wallace, *The Taboo of Subjectivity: Toward a New Science of Consciousness* (New York: Oxford University Press, 2000).

9. See Anthony Ian Jack and Andreas Roepstorff, "Introspection and Cognitive Brain Mapping: From Stimulus-Response to Script-Report," *Trends in Cognitive Sciences* 6 (2002): 333–339.

10. Chris Frith, "How Can We Share Experiences?" *Trends in Cognitive Sciences* 6 (2002): 374.

11. Francisco J. Varela and Jonathan Shear, eds., *The View from Within: First-Person Approaches to the Study of Consciousness* (Thorverton: Imprint Academic, 1999); Natalie Depraz, Francisco J. Varela, and Pierre Vermersch, *On Becoming Aware: A Pragmatics of Experiencing* (Amsterdam: John Benjamins, 2003).

12. Francisco J. Varela, "Neurophenomenology: A Methodological Remedy for the Hard Problem," *Journal of Consciousness Studies* 3 (1996): 330–350. See also Antoine Lutz and Evan Thompson, "Neurophenomenology: Integrating Subjective Experience and Brain Dynamics in Cognitive Neuroscience," *Journal of Consciousness Studies* 10 (2003): 31–52.

13. Lutz et al., "Guiding the Study."

14. On the neurodynamics of epilepsy, see Michel Le Van Quyen et al., "Temporal Patterns in Human Epileptic Activity Are Modulated by Perceptual Discriminations," *Neuroreport* 8 (1997): 1703–1710; Jacques Martinerie et al., "Epileptic Crisis Can Be Anticipated by Non-Linear Analysis," *Nature Medicine* 4 (1998): 1173–1176; Le Van Quyen et al., "Anticipation of Epileptic Seizures." For discussion of the relationship of these neurodynamic studies in relation to issues of cognitive control of epileptic seizure, see Michel Le Van Quyen and Claire Petitmengin, "Neuronal Dynamics and Conscious Experience: An Example of Reciprocal Causation before Epileptic Seizures," *Phenomenology and the Cognitive Sciences* 1 (2002): 169–180. For discussion in relation to theoretical issues about mental causation, see Thompson and Varela, "Radical Embodiment"; Francisco J. Varela and Evan Thompson, "Neural Synchrony and the Unity of Mind: A Neurophenomenological Approach," in *The Unity of Consciousness: Binding, Integration, and Dissociation*, ed. Axel Cleeremans (Oxford: Oxford University Press, 2003), 266–287.

15. See James, *Principles of Psychology*, 191–192.

16. See Wolfgang Köhler, *Gestalt Psychology* (New York: Liveright,

1947), 67–99; Maurice Merleau-Ponty, *Phenomenology of Perception* (London: Routledge, 1962), 3–12.

17. See Russell T. Hurlburt and Christopher L. Heavey, "Telling What We Know: Describing Inner Experience," *Trends in Cognitive Sciences* 9 (2001): 400–403.

18. Richard E. Nisbett and Timothy DeCamp Wilson, "Telling More Than We Can Know: Verbal Reports on Mental Processes," *Psychological Review* 84 (1977): 231–259.

19. Ibid.

20. See B. Alan Wallace, *The Bridge of Quiescence: Experiencing Tibetan Buddhist Meditation* (Chicago: Open Court, 1998); B. Alan Wallace, "The Buddhist Tradition of Samatha: Methods for Refining and Exploring Consciousness," in *View from Within*, ed. Varela and Shear, 175–188; Wallace, *Taboo of Subjectivity*, 103–112.

3. Understandings of Attention and Cognitive Control from Cognitive Neuroscience

1. William James, *The Principles of Psychology* (Cambridge, MA: Harvard University Press, 1981).

2. Ronald A. Rensink, J. Kevin O'Regan, and James J. Clark, "To See or Not to See: The Need for Attention to Perceive Changes in Scenes," *Psychological Science* 8 (1997): 368–373; Daniel J. Simons and Michael S. Ambinder, "Change Blindness: Theory and Consequences," *Current Directions in Psychological Science* 14, no. 1 (1995): 44–48.

3. Richard M. Shiffrin and Walter Schneider, "Controlled and Automatic Human Information Processing: II. Perceptual Learning Automaticity, Attending and a General Theory," *Psychological Review* 84, no. 2 (1977): 127–190; Daniel Kahneman and Anne Treisman, "Changing Views of Attention and Automaticity," in *Varieties of Attention*, ed. Raja Parasuraman and D. Roy Davies (Orlando: Academic Press, 1984), 29–61; Jonathan D. Cohen, Kevin Dunbar, and James L. McClelland, "On the Control of Automatic Processes: A Parallel Distributed Processing Model of the Stroop Effect," *Psychological Review* 97, no. 3 (1990): 332–361.

4. Jeremy M. Wolfe, "Visual Search," in *Attention*, ed. Harold Pashler (Hove, East Sussex: Psychology Press, 1998), 13–74.

5. Anne Treisman and Garry Gelade, "A Feature Integration Theory of Attention," *Cognitive Psychology* 12 (1980): 97–136.

6. John Ridley Stroop, "Studies of Interference in Serial Verbal Reactions," *Journal of Experimental Psychology* 18 (1935): 643–662; Colin M. Macleod, "John Ridley Stroop: Creator of a Landmark Cognitive Task," *Canadian Psychology* 32, no. 3 (1991): 521–524.

7. Colin M. MacLeod, "Half a Century of Research on the Stroop Effect: An Integrative Review," *Psychological Bulletin* 109, no. 2 (1991): 163–203.

8. Earl K. Miller and Jonathan D. Cohen, "An Integrative Theory of Prefrontal Cortex Function," *Annual Review of Neuroscience* 24 (2001): 167–202; Donald T. Stuss and Robert T. Knight, *Principles of Frontal Lobe Function* (New York: Oxford University Press, 2002).

9. Joshua D. Greene et al., "An fMRI Investigation of Emotional Engagement in Moral Judgment," *Science* 293 (2001): 2105–2108; Alan G. Sanfey et al., "The Neural Bases of Economic Decision-Making in the Ultimatum Game," *Science* 300 (2003): 1755–1757.

10. Joshua D. Greene et al., "The Neural Bases of Cognitive Conflict and Control in Moral Judgment," *Neuron* 44, no. 2 (2004): 389–400.

11. Sanfey et al., "Neural Bases."

4. Buddhist Training in Enhanced Cognitive Control

1. William James, *The Principles of Psychology* (1890; New York: Dover, 1950), 1:185.

2. Ibid., 1:424.

3. Ibid., 2:322.

4. William James, *Talks to Teachers on Psychology and to Students on Some of Life's Ideals* (1899; New York: Norton, 1958), 84.

5. Geshe Rabten, *The Mind and Its Functions*, trans. Stephen Batchelor (Mt. Pèlerin: Tharpa Choeling, 1979), 60.

6. Śāntideva, *A Guide to the Bodhisattva Way of Life*, trans. Vesna A. Wallace and B. Alan Wallace (Ithaca: Snow Lion, 1997), 8.1.

7. Quoted in B. Alan Wallace, *The Bridge of Quiescence: Experiencing Tibetan Buddhist Meditation* (Chicago: Open Court, 1998), 118.

8. Asaṅga, *Abhidharma samuccaya of Asaṅga*, ed. Pralhad Pradhan (Santiniketan: Visva-Bharati, 1950), 6.6.

9. James, *Principles of Psychology*, 1:420.

6. Introspection and Mechanism in Mental Imagery

1. Although Stephen Kosslyn spoke on his own at the MIT meeting, his remarks were revised and clarified for this volume in collaboration with Daniel Reisberg and Marlene Behrmann.

2. Moustafa Bensafi et al., "Olfactomotor Activity during Imagery Mimics That during Perception," *Nature Neuroscience* 6 (2003): 1142–1144; Jean Decety and Marc Jeannerod, "Mentally Simulated Movements in Virtual Reality: Does Fitts's Law Hold in Motor Imagery?" *Behavioural Brain Research* 72 (1995): 127–134; Jelena Djordjevic et al., "The Mind's Nose: Effects of Odor and Visual Imagery on Odor Detection," *Psychological Science* 15 (2004): 143–148; Daniel Reisberg, ed., *Auditory Imagery* (Hillsdale, NJ: Erlbaum, 1992).

3. For a review, see Edwin Garrigues Boring, *A History of Experimental Psychology*, 2nd ed. (New York: Appleton-Century-Crofts, 1950).

4. Roger N. Shepard and Lynn A. Cooper, *Mental Images and Their Transformations* (Cambridge, MA: MIT Press, 1982).

5. Stephen M. Kosslyn, Thomas M. Ball, and Brian J. Reiser, "Visual Images Preserve Metric Spatial Information: Evidence from Studies of Image Scanning," *Journal of Experimental Psychology: Human Perception and Performance* 4 (1978): 47–60.

6. Stephen M. Kosslyn, *Image and Mind* (Cambridge, MA: Harvard University Press, 1980).

7. Ronald A. Finke, Steven Pinker, and Martha J. Farah, "Reinterpreting Visual Patterns in Mental Imagery," *Cognitive Science* 13 (1989): 51–78.

8. Deborah Chambers and Daniel Reisberg, "Can Mental Images Be Ambiguous?" *Journal of Experimental Psychology: Human Perception and Performance* 11 (1985): 317–328.

9. Fred W. Mast and Stephen M. Kosslyn, "Visual Mental Images Can Be Ambiguous: Insights from Individual Differences in Spatial Transformation Abilities," *Cognition* 86 (2002): 57–70; Mary A. Peterson et al., "Mental Images Can Be Ambiguous: Reconstruals and Reference-Frame Reversals," *Memory and Cognition* 20 (1992): 107–123; Daniel Reisberg and Deborah Chambers, "Neither Pictures nor Propositions: What Can We Learn from a Mental Image?" *Canadian Journal of Psychology* (1991): 288–302.

10. Stephen M. Kosslyn et al., "Sequential Processes in Image Generation," *Cognitive Psychology* 20 (1988): 319–343.

11. Marlene Behrmann, Stephen M. Kosslyn, and Marc Jeannerod, eds., *The Neuropsychology of Mental Imagery* (New York: Pergamon, 1996); Stephen M. Kosslyn and William L. Thompson, "When Is Early Visual Cortex Activated during Visual Mental Imagery?" *Psychological Bulletin* 129 (2003): 723–746.

7. An Abhidharmic View of Emotional Pathologies and Their Remedies

1. Plato, *The Republic*, 9.580d.

2. For a glimpse of the origins of the Abhidharma, see Rupert Gethin, "The Mātrikās: Memorization, Mindfulness and the List," in *In the Mirror of Memory: Reflections on Mindfulness and Remembrance in Indian and Tibetan Buddhism*, ed. Janet Gyatso (Albany: State University of New York Press, 1992), 149–172.

3. Buddhaghosa wrote commentaries on the seven canonical Abhidharma texts, particularly his famous *Atthasālinî*, a commentary on the *Dhammasaṅgaṇī* section of the Abhidharma. The text I will refer to is Anurudha's *Abhidhammattha Sangaha*, a medieval compilation of Buddhaghosa's work.

4. Louis de la Vallée Poussin, *L'Abhidharmakosha de Vasubandhu* (Brussels: Institut Belge des Hautes Etudes Chinoises, 1971), 1:22. Translation from the French is mine.

5. For a brief but thoughtful discussion of the idea of Buddhism as a psychology, see Luis O. Gomez, "Psychology," in *Encyclopedia of Buddhism*, ed. Robert E. Buswell, Jr. (New York: Macmillan, 2004), 678–692.

6. William James, *The Principles of Psychology* (1891; Cambridge, MA: Harvard University Press, 1983), 185.

7. Ibid., 233.

8. Anguttara 4, 137. Quoted by Louis de la Vallée Poussin, "Notes sur le moment ou *ksana* des bouddhistes," in *Essays on Time*, ed. Hari S. Prasad (Delhi: Sri Satguru, 1991), 69. Translation from the French is mine.

9. James, *Principles of Psychology*, 233.

10. Poussin, "Notes sur le moment," 70–71.

11. Bikkhu Bodhi, ed., A Comprehensive Manual of Abhidharma (Kandy, Sri Lanka: Buddhist Publication Society, 1993), 156.

12. Poussin, "Notes sur le moment," 73.

13. Poussin, L'Abhidharmakosha, 1:30. Translation from the French is mine.

14. Ibid.

15. For an extended discussion of the nature of this sixth type of consciousness, see Herbert V. Guenther, Philosophy and Psychology in the Abhidharma (Berkeley: Shambhala, 1976), 20–30.

16. Walpola Rahula, Le compendium de la super-doctrine d'Asaçga (Paris: Ecole Française d'Extrême Orient, 1971), 17. Although the Theravada Abhidharma does not recognize a distinct store-consciousness, its concept of bhavaçga citta, the life-constituent consciousness, is quite similar. For a view of the complexities of the bhavaçga, see William S. Waldron, The Buddhist Unconscious (London: Routledge Curzon, 2003), 81–87.

17. For more details on these topics, see Waldron, Buddhist Unconscious.

18. They are then said to be conjoined (sampayutta, mtshungs ldan) in that they are simultaneous and have the same sensory basis, the same object, the same aspect or way of apprehending this object, and the same substance (the fact that there can be only one representative of a type of consciousness and mental factor at the same time). See Waldron, Buddhist Unconscious, 205.

19. This list, which is standard in the Tibetan tradition, is a compilation based on Asaçga's Abhidharma-samuccaya. It is not, however, Asaçga's own list, which contains fifty-two items. Rahula, Compendium de la super-doctrine, 7. For a more elaborate discussion of this list, see Geshe Rabten, The Mind and Its Functions (1978; Mt. Pélerin: Rabten Choeling, 1992), and Elizabeth Napper, Mind in Tibetan Buddhism (Ithaca, NY: Snow Lion, 1980). For the lists from some of the other traditions, see Bodhi, Comprehensive Manual, 76–79, and Poussin, L'Abhidharmakosha, 2:150–178.

20. Paul Ricoeur, Oneself as Another (Chicago: University of Chicago Press, 1992).

21. Rahula, Compendium de la super-doctrine, 70. Translation from the French is mine.

22. Jamphel Samphel, "bLo rig[s] gi rnam bzhag nyer mkho kun 'dus blo gsar mig 'byed," 11a, in Napper, *Mind in Tibetan Buddhism*.

23. Bodhi, *Comprehensive Manual*, 80.

24. Ibid., 81.

25. Samphel, "bLo rig[s] gi rnam bzhag," 11b.

26. For a discussion of whether compassion and loving-kindness are emotions, see Georges Dreyfus, "Is Compassion an Emotion? A Cross-Cultural Exploration of Mental Typologies," in *Visions of Compassion: Western Scientists and Tibetan Buddhists Examine Human Nature*, ed. Richard J. Davidson and Anne Harrington (Oxford: Oxford University Press, 2002).

27. Samphel, "bLo rig[s] gi rnam bzhag," 12a.

28. Spinoza, *Ethics*, 4.7.

8. *Emotions from the Perspective of Western Biobehavioral Science*

1. Richard J. Davidson, "Well-Being and Affective Style: Neural Substrates and Biobehavioral Correlates," *Philosophical Transactions of the Royal Society (London)* 359 (2004): 1395–1411.

2. Paul Ekman and Erika L. Rosenberg, eds., *What the Face Reveals* (New York: Oxford University Press, 2005).

3. Peter J. Lang, Margaret M. Bradley, and Bruce N. Cuthbert, "Emotion, Attention, and the Startle Reflex," *Psychological Review* 97 (1990): 377–395.

4. Paul Ekman, "Expression: Panel Discussion," *Annals of the New York Academy of Sciences* 1000 (2003): 266–278.

5. Antoine Lutz et al., "Long-Term Meditators Self-Induce High-Amplitude Synchrony during Mental Practice," *Proceedings of the National Academy of Sciences* 101 (2004): 16369–16373.

6. Antonio R. Damasio, *The Feeling of What Happens* (New York: Harcourt, Brace, 1999).

7. David Watson et al., "Testing a Tripartite Model: I. Evaluating the Convergent and Discriminant Validity of Anxiety and Depression Symptom Scales," *Journal of Abnormal Psychology* 104 (1995): 3–14.

8. Paul Ekman et al., "Buddhist and Psychological Perspectives on Emotions and Well-Being," *Current Directions in Psychological Science* 14 (2005): 59–63.

9. Dalai Lama and Howard C. Cutler, *The Art of Happiness* (New York: Riverhead, 1988).

9. Reflections on "Investigating the Mind," One Year Later

1. For several years the Library of Tibetan Works and Archives under Venerable Achok Rinpoche has organized science instruction for advanced students in the monasteries. Students attend on a volunteer basis, with instruction given by Western scientists. The monks who participate in these science workshops are invited to attend the private meetings organized by Mind and Life in Dharamsala between scientists and the Dalai Lama.

2. Antoine Lutz et al., "Long-Term Meditators Self-Induce High-Amplitude Gamma Synchrony during Mental Practice," *Proceedings of the National Academy of Sciences* 101 (2004): 16369–16373.

3. Harvard researcher Herbert Benson and his Mind/Body Medical Institute must be mentioned here, as well as Jon Kabat-Zinn's seminal work in mindfulness-based stress reduction at the University of Massachusetts. Lengthy bibliographies of research on meditation can be found in Howard R. Jarrell, *International Meditation Bibliography, 1950–1982* (Metuchen, NJ: Scarecrow, 1985), and in Michael Murphy and Steve Donovan, *The Physical and Psychological Effects of Meditation: A Review of Contemporary Research* (Petaluma, CA: Institute of Noetic Sciences, 1999–2004), www.noetic.org/research/medbiblio/index.htm.

4. For information about these studies, see www.sbinstitute.com/research.html.

5. See www.mindandlife.org/confsri04.html.

Index

China (continued)
ent, 13; attitudes toward Tibetan Buddhism in, 16
Christianity, 6, 16, 218, 227
Chu, Steven, 182–183
Clarity. See Attention, clarity of
Cognitive control: of epilepsy, 22–23, 233; vs. attention, 28, 29–33, 34–35, 40; defined, 28; relationship to emotion, 31; relationship to economic decision making, 32; and Buddhism, 38–39, 40, 47–48; of social anxiety disorder, 234
Cognitive neuroscience. See Neuroscience, cognitive
Cohen, Jonathan, 198; on attention and cognitive control, 27–35, 47, 48, 55, 61–62, 63, 65, 232–233; on Buddhist-scientist collaboration, 61–62, 210–211, 229; on role of introspection in psychology, 200, 204; on ethics and science, 208–209, 238; on suffering, 208–209, 238; on experiments, 210–211, 223
Cold Spring Harbor summer courses, 234
Compassion, 39, 159, 176, 185; Dalai Lama on, 6, 15, 110–111, 113, 155, 156–157, 170, 173, 174, 215, 239; and mental imagery/visualization, 72, 76, 78, 108–109; Wallace on, 110–111, 158, 161, 170, 172, 206; as virtuous mental state, 117, 130–131, 134, 135, 139, 144–146; facial expressions associated with, 144–146; brain activity associated with, 147–148, 167, 187; Kahneman on, 157, 160–161; Ricard on, 167–169; Kagan on, 190–194
Consciousness: meta-consciousness, 42, 60, 185, 196, 225, 233–234; as stream, 69–72, 77–78, 123–124; as pure awareness, 73, 91–96, 100–

101, 103–105, 146–147, 196, 201–202; physical basis of, 96–98; as intentional, 125–126, 238; types of, 125–128; afflictive mentation, 127–128; store-consciousness, 127–128, 131–132, 271n16; of emotion, 149; origin in Abhidharma tradition, 181–182. See also Moments of awareness
Cosmology, 15
Creationist science, 236
Cullin, Margaret, 172
Cutler, Howard: The Art of Happiness, 150

Dalai Lama: described at MIT meeting, 3–4, 12–13, 15–16, 91, 180, 198, 214, 223–224, 236; at Dharamsala, 5, 11–12, 16, 181–182, 223, 239, 247, 248–249, 273n1; on compassion, 6, 15, 110–111, 113, 155, 156–157, 170, 173, 174, 215, 239; on happiness, 6, 15, 150, 208, 215, 216–217; Nobel Peace Prize of, 12, 13, 248; on science and technology, 12, 14–16, 214–215, 216, 217–218, 226–227, 228, 241; pacifism of, 13; travels to the West, 13–14; on human values, 15; on China, 16; Stroop test given to, 31; on sensory perception, 48–49, 65, 94–95, 97–98, 187–188, 199–200; on attention, 48–50, 58, 61, 95, 103–104, 222; on aspiration, 49–50; on five mental factors of ascertainment, 49–50; on five omnipresent factors, 49–50; on will (sempa), 49–50; on mental states vs. physical states, 58; on Abhidharma tradition, 61; on meditation, 61, 150, 200, 227, 239, 241; on ethics, 63, 208, 215–217, 218, 225, 239–240; on mental imagery/ visualization, 94–96, 99–100, 103–

Emotion *(continued)*
tion of, 22; relationship to attention, 31–32; relationship to brain activity, 31–32, 113, 141–143, 144, 146–148, 150, 154, 167, 170; anger, 40, 71, 112, 113, 117, 119, 134–135, 136, 137–139, 143, 144, 148–149, 152–155, 156, 157–158, 159, 161–162, 173–174, 190, 210, 225; vs. sensory perception, 42, 120, 121, 125–127; jealousy, 70, 71, 134, 135, 225; hatred, 70, 72–73, 74–75, 110, 162, 217, 225, 238; fear, 70, 112, 113, 143, 144, 148, 154, 158–159, 194, 225; relationship to the self, 70, 130, 136, 137, 138–139, 153, 174; freedom from, 71–73, 74–75, 77–78, 111–112, 117, 135–140, 154, 155–163, 173–174, 225, 232, 238, 263n8; Dalai Lama on, 113, 154–155, 156–157, 174, 217–218, 239; and Buddhist practice, 118, 137–139, 144–148, 149–150, 154, 159–165, 174–176; as virtuous/positive, 128–131, 134–135, 139, 140, 144–146, 158, 166–167, 173, 217–218; as afflictive/negative, 129, 130–131, 132, 134–140, 144, 148–149, 150, 152–163, 166–167, 173–174, 217–218, 225, 249; valenced quality of, 141, 143–144, 147, 148, 221; relationship to behavior, 141–143, 144–146, 149; relationship to sensory perception, 142–143; arousal/strength of, 144, 165, 221; relationship to evolution, 148–149, 152–155, 158, 225; vs. feeling, 149, 158; short-term vs. continuous, 149–150, 155, 239. *See also* Compassion; Loving-kindness
Empathy, 39, 167, 176
Engle, Adam, 10; on conference goals, 4–5; and founding of Mind and Life Institute, 7, 246–247

Enlightenment, the, 190, 240
Epilepsy, 22–23, 233
Ethics: relationship to science, 10, 11, 63, 190–194, 198, 206–207, 208–210, 215, 236–241; and Buddhism, 10, 39, 63–64, 128–131, 137, 139–140, 144, 152, 190, 193–194, 197, 198, 205–206, 208, 209, 213, 215–217, 218, 225, 236–240, 261n2; relationship to happiness, 10, 129–130, 206–208; relationship to knowledge, 10, 198, 199, 205–208, 236–240; moral dilemmas in, 31–32; altruism, 39, 71, 75, 78, 168–169; relationship to quality of life, 63; Dalai Lama on, 63, 208, 215–217, 218, 225, 239–240; value judgments, 69–72, 75, 77, 132, 238; vs. morality, 129–130, 132–133; and motivation, 182–183, 239–240; and education, 238–239
Evolution: and Buddhism, 6, 193–194; and emotion, 148–149, 152–155, 158, 225; and language, 196; and creationism, 236
Executive mental processes, 52–54
Experiments, 220, 227, 228–229; regarding introspection, 19–24, 79–80, 81–90, 105–106, 107, 195, 200–201, 202, 204; regarding attention and cognitive control, 29, 30–32, 33–34, 48, 52–54, 59, 61–63, 165, 211–212; regarding executive mental processes, 52–54; Buddhist-scientist collaboration in design of, 62, 64–65, 98–99, 170–171, 187, 204, 211–212, 213, 223, 228–229; regarding mental imagery, 79–80, 81–90, 98–99, 105–106, 107, 110, 111, 112–114; regarding emotion, 144–148, 152, 166–168, 211–212; on embryos, 181–182; on animals, 182–183; motivation for, 182–183; Lander on, 186–187; regarding

Mental states (continued)
69–71, 73, 75, 77, 94, 95–98, 121,
122, 125–126, 187–188; Plato's
typology, 119; mental factors in,
125–126, 128–135; as intentional,
125–126, 238; primary factor of
awareness in, 125–128; cognitive
functions of, 125–128, 131–132,
134–135, 139; neutral character of,
128–129, 131–133, 158–159; ethical
character of, 128–131, 134–135,
139, 140, 144–146, 158–159, 166–
167, 173; afflictive character of, 129,
130–131, 134–140, 144, 148–149,
150, 152–163, 166–167, 173–174;
vs. character traits, 149–150, 152,
154, 162, 186
Meyer, David, 47; on "multitasking addiction disorder" (MAD), 51–54, 56;
on experiments regarding attention,
59, 60; on Buddhist-scientist collaboration, 64–65
Mezirow, Jack, 238–239
Mind and Life Institute: sponsorship of
MIT conference by, 4–6, 7–9, 16–
17; founding of, 5, 7, 19; and Engle,
7, 246–247; and Varela, 7–8, 19,
228, 246–247; funding of Buddhist-
scientist collaboration by, 232–234;
Summer Research Institute, 233,
234–236, 246, 250; partnership with
Dalai Lama, 245, 246–247; history
and activities, 245–250; publications
of, 262n5; Web site, 262n6
Mind/Body Medical Institute,
273n3
Mindfulness, 55–56, 172, 234, 273n3;
relationship to attention, 41–42,
112, 133, 138, 185, 233; Ricard on,
159–160
Minsky, Marvin, 186
Moments of awareness: in attention,
33–34, 42–43, 56–58; duration of,

33–34, 42–43, 56–58, 101, 124, 231;
in Abhidharma tradition, 121, 122,
123–125, 126–128, 139. See also
Consciousness
Motivation, 199; for experimentation,
182–183; Dalai Lama on, 182–183,
239–240; and ethics, 182–183, 239–
240
Multitasking, 51–56, 185;
"multitasking addiction disorder"
(MAD), 51–54, 56
Music, 197

Nalanda University, 40, 228
Neurophenomenology, 7–8, 19–24,
220, 228, 229–230
Neuroplasticity, 249–250
Neuroscience, cognitive, 208–209,
248; and Varela, 7–8, 19–20, 22–23,
229–230; Frith on, 21–22; study of
attention in, 27–35, 56; taxonomy of
mental functions in, 88
Nirvana, 120
Nisbett, Richard E., 23

"Online compulsive disorder" (OCD),
54, 55
Openness, 12, 181–182, 226–227
Orientalism, 8, 262n7

Pain control, 80, 108, 110
Patience, 162–163
Patrul, Rinpoche, 162–163
Physics, 15, 93–94, 196–197, 228;
super-string theory, 201; quantum
mechanics, 201, 248–249; imper-
sonal perspective in, 203
Placebo effects, 34–35
Plato: on three parts of the soul, 119;
on ethics, 207
Pleasure, 70–71, 77–78; in
Abhidharma tradition, 125, 126,
128, 130, 132, 136–137; in neurosci-

ence, 144, 145, 163–164, 221; relationship to happiness, 150, 163–164; hedonic treadmill, 150, 163–164
Popularity of MIT conference, 189, 194, 223–224
Prefrontal cortex, 31–32, 147–148
Pride, 70, 71, 134, 135
Problem solving, 204
Proust, Marcel, 196
Psychology, 208–209; and Buddhism, 6–7, 15, 21, 117, 118, 228; role of introspection in, 19–24, 200–201, 204, 224, 228; Gestalt psychology, 21, 23; phenomenological psychology, 21, 23, 185; cognitive psychology, 50–51; and mental images/visualization, 102–103; hedonic treadmill, 150, 163–164; psychophysics, 200

Rabten, Geshe, 164
Reality monitoring, 101–102
Reality vs. delusion, 10, 24, 153; regarding emotions, 69–73, 77–78, 173–174; regarding phenomenal world/material things, 69–73, 101–102, 120, 121, 205–207, 238; regarding the self, 70–71, 72, 77–78, 93, 113, 121, 127–128, 135, 137, 138–139, 166, 174, 186, 199–200, 238
Reason, 188, 205, 226–227, 238–239; Dalai Lama on, 156–157, 199–200, 227, 239, 241; and problem solving, 204
Reisberg, Daniel, 91, 94, 233; on introspection, 79–90; on pure awareness, 93; on mental imaging/visualization, 102–103, 104, 110; on creative problem solving, 110
Renaissance, 190
Ricard, Matthieu, 9, 151, 183–184; on mental imagery in Buddhism, 69–78, 92–93, 95, 99, 101–102, 105,

107, 108–109, 112, 222; on pure awareness, 73, 91–93, 104–105; on pain control, 110; relationship with Davidson, 144–146, 152, 168, 170–171, 172, 184, 212, 230–231, 232, 263n8; on afflictive emotions, 152–153, 161, 162–163; on training, 159, 176, 212; on freedom and self-control, 159–160; on mindfulness, 159–160; on compassion, 167–169; on loving-kindness, 167–169; on attachment, 173; on meditation and child development, 175; on ethics and knowledge, 207; on suffering, 207; on Buddhist-scientist collaboration, 212, 263n8
Ricoeur, Paul, 129
RNA, 11, 184

Said, Edward, on orientalism, 263n7
samadhi, 202, 205, 213
Santa Barbara Institute, 233
Sariputta, 57–58
Scharmer, Claus Otto, 224–225
Science: scientific method, 4, 7–8; as dominant in modern society, 4, 9; Christianity in conflict with, 6; relationship to ethics, 10, 11, 63, 190–194, 198, 206–207, 208–210, 215, 236–241; Dalai Lama on, 12, 14–16, 214–215, 216, 217–218, 226–227, 228, 241; and humanities, 16–17; and emotion, 141–150, 151, 165, 166–167, 168; motivation of scientists, 182–183; new questions in, 185; relationship to happiness, 210; and religious commitments, 236. *See also* Brain activity; Buddhist-scientist collaboration; Experiments; Neuroscience, cognitive; Psychology
Self, the: relationship to emotion, 70, 130, 136, 137, 138–139, 153, 174;

Self, the *(continued)*
reality vs. delusion regarding, 70–71, 72, 77–78, 93, 113, 121, 127–128, 135, 137, 138–139, 166, 174, 186, 199–200, 238; Dalai Lama on, 113, 174, 199–200; in non-Buddhist Indian traditions, 170
Sensory perception: vs. mental states, 42, 48–49, 51, 70–71, 77, 94–95, 96–97, 100–102, 104–107, 109–112, 142–143, 187–188; and Buddhism, 48–49, 65, 69–78, 94–95, 97–98, 120, 121, 125–127, 131–132, 136–137, 187–188, 199–200; Dalai Lama on, 48–49, 65, 94–95, 97–98, 187–188, 199–200; vs. mental imaging/visualization, 88–89; in Abhidharma tradition, 120, 121, 125–127; and language, 196
shamatha (mental quiescence), 233
Shantideva: *A Guide to the Bodhisattva Way of Life*, 40
Sharp, Phillip, 11, 12
Shechen monastery, 9
Shepard, Roger, 82
Simon, Herbert, 157, 204
Social anxiety disorder, 234
Spinoza, Benedict de, 137
Stress reduction, 233, 273n3
Stroop test, 30–31
Subjective experience, 19–24; relationship to brain activity, 7, 8, 19, 20, 22–23, 24, 37, 43–45, 57–58, 88, 96–98, 106, 107, 111–113, 124, 140, 141–143, 144–148, 152, 183–184, 185, 187, 194, 195, 197, 219–220, 226, 230, 233, 234, 235; Varela on, 7–8, 19–20, 22; relationship to behavior, 8, 20, 23, 24, 28, 29–30, 32, 34–35, 37, 43–45, 81, 111–112, 114, 141–142, 144–148, 149, 169–171, 197, 202–203, 205–206, 221, 223, 235; James on, 20–21, 37, 64; Frith

on, 21–22. *See also* Meditation; Mental imagery/visualization; Mental states
Suffering: causes of, 10, 40, 70–72, 75, 130–131, 134–135, 136, 166–167, 173–174, 207–209, 211, 215–217; freedom from, 71–73, 75, 77, 108–109, 130–131, 134, 167–168, 183, 189, 207–208, 215–217, 221, 238; Wallace on, 158–159, 173–174; Dalai Lama on, 208, 215–216; Four Noble Truths, 215–217
Sufism, 16
Sutra system, 97

Theravada Buddhism, 9, 21, 120, 124, 271n16
Thompson, Evan, 198; on first-person vs. third-person perspective, 202–203, 219–220, 226; on Varela, 229–230; on Buddhist claims, 231
Thurman, Robert, 13
Tibetan Buddhism, 227, 228, 232; as focus of MIT conference, 5; idealized attitudes toward, 8, 13–14; Western attitudes toward, 8, 13–14, 222–223; modernization movement in, 14–15; Chinese attitudes toward, 16; and attention, 34, 39–41, 44, 54–55, 60–61, 103–104; and emotion, 118–119, 145; and child development, 174–176; and scientific experiments, 211–212; and Tibetan culture, 223; Library of Tibetan Works and Archives, 273n1
Tibet House, 13
Training, 150, 157, 238; of attention, 22, 34, 37–45, 47, 51, 54, 56–57, 59, 60–61, 73–77, 95, 98–99, 103–104, 106, 112, 184, 187, 213, 230; vs. lack of training, 33–34, 40, 41–42, 43–44, 98–99, 102–103, 106, 111, 124, 146–147, 149, 156, 170–171,